ALTERNATIVE MEDICINE

PRACTICES, HEALTH BENEFITS AND CONTROVERSIES

HEALTH CARE ISSUES, COSTS AND ACCESS

ALTERNATIVE MEDICINE

PRACTICES, HEALTH BENEFITS AND CONTROVERSIES

KENNETH R. CARTER
AND
GEORGE E. MURPHY
EDITORS

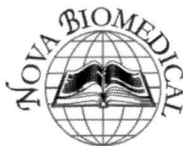

NOVA BIOMEDICAL

New York

NOTICE TO THE READER

The Publisher has taken reasonable care in the preparation of this book, but makes no expressed or implied warranty of any kind and assumes no responsibility for any errors or omissions. No liability is assumed for incidental or consequential damages in connection with or arising out of information contained in this book. The Publisher shall not be liable for any special, consequential, or exemplary damages resulting, in whole or in part, from the readers' use of, or reliance upon, this material. Any parts of this book based on government reports are so indicated and copyright is claimed for those parts to the extent applicable to compilations of such works.

Independent verification should be sought for any data, advice or recommendations contained in this book. In addition, no responsibility is assumed by the publisher for any injury and/or damage to persons or property arising from any methods, products, instructions, ideas or otherwise contained in this publication.

This publication is designed to provide accurate and authoritative information with regard to the subject matter covered herein. It is sold with the clear understanding that the Publisher is not engaged in rendering legal or any other professional services. If legal or any other expert assistance is required, the services of a competent person should be sought. FROM A DECLARATION OF PARTICIPANTS JOINTLY ADOPTED BY A COMMITTEE OF THE AMERICAN BAR ASSOCIATION AND A COMMITTEE OF PUBLISHERS.

Additional color graphics may be available in the e-book version of this book.

Library of Congress Cataloging-in-Publication Data

Library of Congress Control Number: 2012939742

ISBN: 978-1-62257-106-2

Published by Nova Science Publishers, Inc. † New York

CONTENTS

PREFACE

Complementary and alternative are terms used to describe a number of products, practices, and systems that are not part of mainstream (conventional, standard, or Western) medicine. They can include methods like herbs and dietary supplements, body movement, spiritual approaches, pills, extracts, creams and ointments. In this book, the authors present research from across the globe in the study of some practices, health benefits and controversies associated with alternative medicine. Topics include reflexology therapy as a form of manual pressure applied mostly to the feet; alternative therapies for children with attention-deficit/hyperactivity disorder; alternative medicine combined with integrative medicine to treat chronically ill patients; and complementary medicine use in pediatric inflammatory bowel disease, cancer, and epilepsy.

Chapter 1 - The chapter introduces images, their characteristics, habitual contexts and cognitive functions. The following sections provide a review of studies that focus on guided imagery as a therapeutic option in the domain of medicine. The special themes dealt with include the effects of guided imagery on coping, on reducing stress, on symptoms due to different diseases and the administered treatments, on pain, on healing and on different parameters of the immune system. The final section deals with guided imagery in the clinical setting, describing in detail the Kreitler method of guided imagery, presenting its operational procedure and theoretical rationale. Concluding remarks refer to advantages and risks of applying guided imagery.

Chapter 2 - The use of complementary and alternative therapies, even in western industrialised countries with well developed conventional health care systems, ranges from 10-52%. Annual expenditure on complementary and alternative medicine (CAM) in the UK alone is estimated to be in excess of £1.6 billion. Despite this extensive use, complementary and alternative therapies have recently come under scrutiny in terms of their safety and efficacy, particularly in relation to claims made by practitioners. To date, robust scientific evidence for health benefit has been lacking for many alternative therapies, but despite this they remain popular.

Reflexology therapy is a form of sophisticated manual pressure applied most typically to the feet. It is one of the top six complementary and alternative therapies purchased. It is distinct from general massage due to two key therapeutic claims. First, that distinct areas on the feet correspond to specific internal organs within the body. Second, that massage to these discreet areas affects the haemodynamic status of the referred or 'mapped' organs in the body.

This chapter will describe and discuss in detail the basis for these haemodynamic theories by reviewing the original work of William H Fitzgerald and Eunice Ingham. The chapter will finish by describing the available contemporary evidence to support these theories and discusses the challenge of proving specific treatment effects in CAM in this current era of evidence-based medicine.

Chapter 3 - According to the systematic reviews the data on the safety, effectiveness and efficacy and long-term use of stimulant medications for paediatric Attention-Deficit/Hyperactivity Disorder (AD/HD) is conflicting. Uncertainty still surrounds the balance of risks and benefits of long-term drug treatment. Current evidence strongly points to significant parental concerns about exposing their children to psychopharmacological interventions. This appears to be the case despite the evidence base for the use of stimulant medications. Children with AD/HD who are treated with stimulants often show side-effects. Across studies, the most frequently examined adverse effects of stimulant medications have been appetite suppression, weight loss, sleep disturbances, irritability, stomach aches, headaches, rashes, nausea, fatigue and occasionally the development or aggravation of tics. Cardiovascular effects and reductions in growth velocity have also been reported. Controversy over the safety and appropriateness of stimulant treatment has led to increased parental anxiety and the increased use of complementary and alternative medicine (CAM) therapies. Many parents prefer to find more natural treatments for their children with AD/HD. In general, parents seek CAM therapies for their children because a particular allopathic treatment was considered ineffective, dissatisfaction with conventional medicine, fear of drug adverse effects and a need for more personal attention for their children. As a result of this controversy, CAM therapies are sought more often by parents who have children with developmental and behavioural disorders such as AD/HD, than with any other condition. The following chapter outlines the variety of CAM therapies available for paediatric AD/HD.

Chapter 4 - The increasing incidence of chronic illness and the popularity of integrative medicine approaches as treatment modalities require that we better understand the meaning that chronically ill patients attribute to their illness and treatment experience. This paper is based on a phenomenological study that sought to understand how nine chronically ill patients perceived their experience of living with their illnesses and receiving treatment at an integrative medicine clinic situated in an urban centre in Canada. Participants' accounts of how they experienced their health and illness were framed as contrasts between their past and present selves. Their experience of their relationships with and care received from providers at the integrative clinic was framed against the backdrop of their experiences in conventional medicine contexts. The findings indicate that participants' illnesses disrupted their life and sense of self. Declining health and influence of members in their social milieu were impetuses for joining the clinic, where participants developed enriched relationships with clinicians. These relationships allowed them to feel cared for and empowered. Following treatments at the clinic, participants experienced improvements in their health status, a return to their old or renewed sense of self, and hope for the future. We provide rich data from the participants' interviews, and we consider the implications of living with and receiving treatment for chronic illness.

Chapter 5 - Following diagnosis with a chronic incurable illness, such as Inflammatory Bowel Disease (IBD), children and their families often face uncertainty and worries. These include concerns about the need for standard medical therapies, and the potential side-effects of these treatments. Further, the available drugs have variable benefits and may not always assist adequately in the management of the child's disease.

Consequently, many parents and families look to other options, including complementary and alternative medicines (CAM) as ways to help their child's condition.

Chapter 6 - "Complementary" and "Alternative" are terms used to describe a number of products, practices, and systems that are not part of mainstream (conventional, standard, or Western) medicine. They can include methods like herbs and dietary supplements, body movement, spiritual approaches, pills, extracts, and creams and ointments. Some are done by a person with extensive formal education and training (art therapy), while others may be recommended by the person who is selling the product in a store or on the Internet (colon therapy) or needles acupuncture) to no-touch "energy work" (reiki). Some are time-consuming or expensive (rigid diets or treatments in another country); others are fairly cheap and easy to use (vitamins or homeopathy). Some can be done at home on your own (meditation) and others require another person to give them (massage). Some almost never cause harm, while others can be dangerous and cause deaths.

Chapter 7 - Throughout the world, many people use complementary and alternative medicine (CAM) to treat epilepsy. One common CAM used is herbal medicine.

Although many plant ingredients are used in modern medications and some appear to have anticonvulsant properties, there are no evidence-based clinical studies that any control epileptic seizures. Difficulties with plant studies arise because concentrations of active principles can vary according to growing conditions. Some are also known to act on the cytochrome p450 system to alter plasma anti-epileptic drug (AED) levels, possibly detrimentally. Literature on other CAMs used in epilepsy is readily available.

Acupuncture studies in animals reveal antiepileptic effects and are likely secondary to altering neurotransmission. Prayer, music, and relaxation techniques are also frequently used CAMs. Vitamins and minerals can help prevent some secondary effects of AEDs. Ketogenic and Atkins diets have been found to be useful evidence-based CAM treatments in refractory epilepsies of children and adults. Surveys from Asia, Europe, and the United States have shown that 35 to 72% of patients with severe or refractory neurological disorders use CAM, although many do not report it to their physicians.

This percentage is similar for patients with epilepsy, who commonly switch to CAM or combine CAM with prescribed medications. The chance that CAM will be used for an illness appears related to experience with CAM use in the past and a belief in the safety of CAM use. Patients with advanced education degrees beyond upper school appear to have a higher prevalence of CAM use.

Commonly patients think that CAMs are safer, more "natural", and lack secondary adverse effects. However, most CAM use is likely precipitated by dissatisfaction with failed evidence-based medical treatments, lack of access to or unavailability of AEDs, inadequate education about epilepsy, insufficient resources, and cultural beliefs. Cultures which believe in diseases caused by "the supernatural" use traditional medicine/CAM as initial therapy rather than of modern medical therapies.

CAM use to treat epilepsy has five possible outcomes to the patient. First, their effect is neutral or not harmful and/or they do not interact with an AED or other modern epilepsy treatments. Second, their effect is detrimental to the patient because of direct effects or undesired interactions. Third, they are not effective as an AED, but they do promote general health.

Fourth, their effect is unknown, and, therefore, most likely risky. Fifth, they are effective as an AED. CAM use in epilepsy patients often is related to non-adherence to evidence-based AED treatment. Because of the wide range of CAM effects, patients and medical providers need to discuss openly the use of CAM in the treatment of epilepsy. A comprehensive epilepsy education program is needed initially to change non-adherent behaviors and to close the treatment gap for epilepsy.

This must go hand-in-hand with improved access to resources and treatment. At the same time, clinical translational research needs to be promoted to determine newer specific and adjuvant therapies for epilepsy, some of which may prove to be CAMs currently in use.

In: Alternative Medicine
Editors: Kenneth R. Carter and George E. Murphy

ISBN 978-1-62257-106-2
©2012 Nova Science Publishers, Inc.

Chapter 1

GUIDED IMAGERY: A PSYCHOLOGICAL TOOL IN THE SERVICE OF HEALTH PSYCHOLOGY

Shulamith Kreitler

School of Psychological Sciences, Tel-Aviv University, Tel-Aviv, Israel

ABSTRACT

The first part of the chapter introduces images, their characteristics, habitual contexts and cognitive functions. The following sections provide a review of studies that focus on guided imagery as a therapeutic option in the domain of medicine. The special themes dealt with include the effects of guided imagery on coping, on reducing stress, on symptoms due to different diseases and the administered treatments, on pain, on healing and on different parameters of the immune system. The final section deals with guided imagery in the clinical setting, describing in detail the Kreitler method of guided imagery, presenting its operational procedure and theoretical rationale. Concluding remarks refer to advantages and risks of applying guided imagery.

IMAGERY: CHARACTERISTICS AND CONTEXTS

The term imagery has come to denote a whole set of kinds of images that have been identified in different contexts and with different methods. Thus, there are references in the literature to mental images, sensory images, memory images, thought images, eidetic images, symbolic images, dream images, afterimages, déjà vu images, and last but not least, hallucinations of different kinds (Roeckelein, 2004). The diversity in terms may serve as evidence for the ubiquity of images and for the multiple roles they fulfill in different domains.

Guided imagery (GI) is imagery used in a particular way and for a particular purpose. Basically it is imagery and as such it is a specific kind of cognitive act that is often called imagining, visualizing, picturing, or reconstructing in the mind's eye. Imagery – both in the sense of images and the processes of constructing images - forms part of the cognitive system or faculty of imagination. In defining GI we will first distinguish it from other constructs with which it has often been confused.

GI is sometimes considered as a kind of hypnosis. There are indeed some features that these two techniques may share, such as the use of imagery and application in regard to bodily states. Moreover, GI is sometimes used as a method for the induction of hypnosis (Gafner, 2010) or in the course of hypnosis (e.g., Zachariae, Bjerring and Arendt-Nielsen, 2007). However, GI is not hypnosis. The main differences are that hypnosis is based on involving a deeper and more comprehensive change in consciousness as well as a longer and more complex induction procedure. Further, hypnosis does not rely exclusively on the use of imagery and it may be used also for psychologically-based disorders.

Another distinction that needs to be made is between GI and relaxation techniques. GI may be used for relaxation but it remains only one of its applications. Further, relaxation techniques rely mostly on the use of means other than imagery, such as muscle contractions.

GI is characterized by applying images as a major component. Imagery has often been considered as part of perception and there are investigators who propound the so-called pictorial approach to imagery (Kosslyn, 1994; Shepard and Metzler, 1983). Indeed, images resemble percepts in having sensory features which make them into concrete constructs, and in referring to specific concrete objects or situations. But they differ from percepts in that the objects or situations to which they refer are not physically present and in being mostly less vivid than percepts. However the major feature distinguishing images from percepts is that images are under cognitive control in their occurrence, contents, and appearance.

Recent neurological research has provided additional confirmation for the conclusion that images differ from percepts. While imagining and perceiving have similar neural substrates, they manifest different network dynamics. Thus, for seen objects there was a clear posterior–anterior gradient along the ventral visual stream, whereas for imagined objects there was an opposite gradient. Further, in all regions along the visual stream there was more similarity between responses to all imagined objects than between the perceived ones (Lee, Kravitz and Baker, 2012).

Characteristics of images. As noted, imagery is a part of imagination, which can be considered as a subsystem of cognition. Hence, images are a particular form of cognitive contents. There are two major characteristics of images. The first characteristic is their form, which is concrete. The *concreteness of images* is manifested in two ways: the images refer to objects or situations that exist or could exist in external reality and the images are endowed with sensory characteristics. Although most discussions of imagery focus mainly or exclusively upon the visual mode, images in other sensory modes are just as common and significant psychologically (Newton, 1982). Thus, in addition to visual imagery that refers to brightness (or light), color, form (or shapes), and movement, there is auditory, olfactory, gustatory, haptic or tactile (touch), thermal and kinaesthetic (motor) imagery, as well as imagery based on internal senses, such as pain, balance and acceleration, sexuality, and pressure (e.g., Segal and Fusella, 1971; Reisberg, 1992; Klatzky, Lederman, and Matula, 1991; Jeannerod, 1994; Bensafi *et al.*, 2003).

Despite the fact that images are usually categorized so that they correspond to one of the senses, two deviations from this rule need to be noted. First, it is possible to have an image that consists of combined referencesto two or more sensory modes, such as an image that is both haptic and auditory. The second deviation consists of synesthetic imagery, namely, imagery that may apparently be evoked by stimuli of one sensory mode but may consist of an experience in another sensory mode. In the original sense, synesthesia refers to images triggered by perceptually presented stimuli (e.g., sweet taste evoked by sounds), but it is possible to have synesthetic images in response to stimuli that are themselves images (i.e., both the sweetness and the sounds are images).

The second characteristic of images is *cognitive malleability*. This means that images may be shaped, constructed, combined with other images or constructs, transformed and otherwise manipulated so as to serve adequately one's purpose or vision. In order to clarify the difference between images and percepts Pylyshin (1999) emphasized that images are "cognitively penetrable", by which he meant that changes may be inserted or implanted in the image so that it is changed structurally in order to conform to functional requirements. It is this characteristic of images that enables to turn them into "guided" images.

Contexts of images. Images occur spontaneously in a variety of contexts. Major among these are night dreams and daydreams. Another common context is altered states of consciousness, including trance and mystical states, the passages between wakefulness and sleep (hypnagogia and hypnopompia), and those induced by various physiological and psychological means, such as alcohol, opiates, or psychoactive drugs both of the traditional type and the more modern hallucinogens. A special context consists of meditation, prayer, different kinds of Yoga (e.g., dream Yoga), hypnosis and lucid dreaming. A further context is physiological states induced by fever, nitrogen narcosis (deep diving), diseases such as temporal lobe epilepsy or delirium, infections such as meningitis, as well as deprivation of sleep, of food (fasting), of oxygen or of sensation (sensory deprivation). Psychopathologies form another context in which images occur, for example, in psychoses or as hallucinations that may or may not be accompanied by psychosis. Finally, there is evidence about images that occur under exceptional circumstances, such as peak experiences, traumatic accidents, child delivery, or extraordinary excitement (Kreitler, 2009).

Images in the domain of cognition. Images have been found to fulfill a basic role in different contexts of cognition. Paivio (1971) was one of the first investigators who emphasized the major role of verbal images in thinking. In recent years a body of research has accumulated demonstrating the role of images in creative thinking in the sciences and the arts (Antonietti and Colombo, 2011; Palmiero, Cardi, and Belardinelli, 2011; West, 2009), in problem solving, particularly of novel problems (Clement, 2008), in associations (Newton, 1993), memory (Tom and Tversky, 2012), learning (Moore and Carlson, 2012), and consciousness (Newton, 1993). Notably, the processes based on imagery were found often to precede or function iteratively with the more formal abstract processes in problem solving (Clement, 2008). In all cases the involvement of imagery functions as a facilitating factor, improving the performance of the cognitive act and raising the level of the output. It should however be noted that producing images is in itself a cognitive act that uses cognitive resources. It was shown that when pictures were used in a learning set, they enhanced comprehension and reduced cognitive load in the learners. But when the learners were requested to generate images on their own, their cognitive load increased and comprehension decreased, probably because they had fewer cognitive resources available for cognitive processing (Schwamborn, Thillmann, Opfermann and Leutner, 2011).

Some interim conclusions. The reported observations and studies support several conclusions that may help in conceptualizing the nature and role of GI. One conclusion is that images are a natural and common tool that is well known to many people from a variety of contexts. Hence the use of imagery in GI would not be a surprising or unusual event for most participants. Another conclusion is that images are an important component of the cognitive system, involved in the performance of cognitive acts of various kinds. A third conclusion is that images seem to be involved in cognitive acts based on standard reasoning (e.g., problem solving in mathematics) as well as creative thinking and art production. In other words, imagery is related both to conscious and unconscious cognition.

GI IN DOMAINS WITH RELEVANCE FOR HEALTH

Introductory remarks. GI in one form or another is one of the world's most ancient forms of healing (Achtenberg, 1985). It is also one of the most common methods, practiced by a great number of people in most cultures, including the Western world (Heinschel, 2002). About a decade ago it has been reported that at least 10 million Americans admit to using GI for coping with life and health stresses of different kinds (O'Donnell et al., 2002). This should not be surprising because GI seems to have many advantages: it is cheap, it is constantly available, it is accessible to everyone, it can be practiced on one's own without the intervention of other agents, it has apparently no negative effects, it is "respectable" in the sense that it belongs to body-mind practices and not to any mystic sects, and last but not least , its applications appear to be broad-ranged, including sports, physical disorders, psychological symptoms, distress and everyday-life problems.

However, the widespread use of GI may be related to two major shortcomings. One is the absence of a standard procedure of practicing GI. It is sometimes restricted only to the use of visualization, at other times it may rely on using only other sensory images exclusively or in addition to the visual images. Sometimes specific images are used, for example, images that refer to particular contents, at other times the individual is encouraged to use any images he or she wants as long as they are images. Sometimes words are used in addition to images, at other times no words are used. In some cases GI is completely self-guided, at other times there may be a guide who accompanies the process or the individual may use an audio-tape. A special variety of GI is "interactive GI" whereby a guide or mentor helps in shaping the images in the course of the GI session itself. Further, in many contexts the GI is used together with other practices, such as music therapy, breathing exercises, lucid dreaming, yoga and meditation or even interchangeably with practices of relaxation, drawings, dream interpretations, fantasy explorations, mindfulness, meditation and hypnosis (Foote, 1996; Kabat-Zinn, 1990). This broad-ranged use of GI, without a standard set of application guidelines, may have contributed to the second shortcoming which is the limited empirical basis for supporting conclusions about the functions of GI in medicine and for promoting health and well-being in general. Indeed, there are many studies in this domain but it may often be difficult to compare them so as to reach an evidence-based conclusion supported by the common criteria.

GI as a therapeutic option in medicine. Different studies report that patients use or request the availability of services related to GI in the context of alternative therapies. Thus, for example, frequent uses of GI were reported for adolescent asthma patients (Cotton, Luberto and Tsevat, 2011), pediatric cancer patients (Kemper and Wornham, 2001) and breast cancer patients (Ben-Arye et al., 2009). Patients in these groups emphasized their expectations that GI would help them to alleviate symptoms, such as nausea, fatigue, pain and breathing difficulties. There is evidence about frequent use of GI in a variety of medical setups, such as diagnostic imaging in radiology departments (Puchalski, 2000), hospice wards in the State of Washington in the US (45% used GI) (Kozak et al., 2009), or pediatric pain management service (49% used GI) (Lin, Lee, Kemper and Berde, 2005). A National Health Interview Survey conducted with a sample of 2262 adults diagnosed with cancer (representing 14.3 million cancer survivors in the US) about the uses of complementary medicine showed that 1.6% of the men and 4.5% of the women used GI, whereby there were 5 complementary medicine practices that were used more frequently and 8 more rarely. People diagnosed with lymphoma or prostate cancer, or patients suffering from depression or fatigue tended to use GI more often than others (Fouladbakhsh and Stommel, 2010).

GI as a means for coping. The beneficial uses of imagination for overcoming fears and physical hardship have been discussed by such diverse authors as Hilgard (1977), Frankl (1970), Winnicott (1971), and Singer and Singer (1990). Clark (1998) reported how the use of imagination by children with various chronic diseases helped them to cope with their fears of the illness and the treatments. Brewin, Dalgleish and Joseph (1996) demonstrated that accessing memories of traumatic events via images complements the verbally accessible memories and in this manner promotes a more complete resolution of the trauma. Others emphasized the role of images as a means of detachment that enables a better resolution of the problem one faces (Lynn, Pintar and Rhue, 1997). Another likely benefit of imagery for coping is the possibility it affords to try out different solutions and options in an imaginary world, without being limited by various reality constraints (Goldstein and Russ, 2001; Singer and Singer, 1990). Further research shows that imagination is a useful means for integrating problem-focused and emotion-focused coping in the interests of better emotion regulation (Taylor et al., 1998).

These properties of imagery have been utilized in interactive GI for assisting individuals to overcome fear of flying, and prepare for stressful situations, such as public speaking or appearing in a courtroom (Gary, 2011). It is likely that the contribution of GI to coping underlies also the reported effects of GI in sports. A study with varsity athletes showed that imagery predicted mental toughness and that motivational general-mastery imagery was the strongest single predictor for all dimensions of mental toughness (Mattie and Munroe-Chandler, 2012). High scores in mental imagery were related also to motor performance in elite and novice athletes, contributing especially to complex motor acts requiring efficiency in the use of flexible strategies, that enable adjusting to the particular problems encountered (Moreau, Mansy-Dannay, Clerc and Guerrién, 2011).

Also in the medical framework GI is used for helping patients cope better with the problems posed by the illness and the treatments. Three brief case studies presented by Rossman (2002) illustrate how GI was used for helping cancer patients to construct a more comprehensive view of their treatment course, find strength to continue along this course, or make serious decisions concerning their treatment. GI has also been used for improving coping with pain. An intervention involving GI and skills instruction resulted in increased pain tolerance in university students performing a cold pressor task. Notably, the intervention did not affect the pain threshold, which indicates that it facilitated pain tolerance without affecting the pain experience itself (Berg, Snyder and Hamilton, 2008).

GI as a modulator of stress. Stress was shown to be a factor that is involved in the occurrence of disease and its course. Several studies highlight the function of GI in modulating stress. A study done with nursing students showed that GI reduced their stress and improved the performance level of intramuscular injections they were taught to do (Suk, Oh and Kil, 2006). Another study with shift-working nurses dealt with reducing the stress caused by deviating from regular circadian rhythms (Rider, Floyd and Kirkpatrick, 1985). The intervention which consisted in listening on a daily basis to a tape providing music, progressive muscle relaxation and GI resulted in significant decreases of the mean levels of the circadian amplitude of adrenal corticosteroids (viz. "stress hormones") as well as the circadian temperature rhythms.

GI proved effective also in reducing stress in centrifuge training in pilots, cosmonauts and astronauts. At three measurement points (before intervention, after it and after the centrifuge training) those who underwent GI had lower anxiety, lower tension and lower heart rate (decrease in low frequency components and increase in high frequency components) than those who underwent music intervention (Jing et al., 2011).

Post-traumatic stress disorder represents a different kind of stress. A study with adolescents in postwar Kosovar showed that a 12 session GI intervention reduced their stress symptoms as assessed by the Harvard Trauma Questionnaire (Gordon et al., 2008). The intervention was conducted by trained and supervised school teachers and the reduction in stress persisted until 3 months following the intervention.

A pre-surgery intervention that included GI reduced the stress and improved the wound healing in surgical patients who underwent elective laparoscopic cholecystectomy (Broadbent et al., 2012). Another study focused on the effects of a 4-week pilot Interactive GI intervention on stress-reduction in overweight Latino adolescents. It was assumed that since chronic stress with relative hypercortisolism has been associated with metabolic disease risk, reducing the stress of these adolescents may reduce their disease risk. Moderate to high reductions in cortisol were attained (Weigensberg et al., 2009). A study with pregnant women focused on reducing stress assessed at four time points before and after the intervention in terms of self-reported relaxation on a visual analog scale, state anxiety, endocrine parameters indicating hypothalamic-pituitary-adrenal axis (cortisol and ACTH) and sympathetic-adrenal-medullary system activity (norepinephrine and epinephrine), as well as cardiovascular responses (heart rate, systolic and diastolic blood pressure). GI proved to be more effective in enhancing relaxation than progressive muscle relaxation or passive relaxation techniques (Urech et al., 2010).

GI effects on alleviating different physical symptoms related to the disease or the treatment. Applying GI singly or in combination with some other relaxation techniques has been used widely for alleviating physical disease- or treatment-related symptoms.

An early study used GI for affecting postoperative responses of pediatric surgical patients (Lambert, 1996). The children of the experimental group were taught GI which included suggestions for a favorable postoperative course. Significantly lower postoperative pain ratings and shorter hospital stays were reported for children in the experimental group than in the control group. State anxiety was decreased in the GI group and increased postoperatively in the control group.

The three following studies found no postoperative effects for GI. In one study (Haase et al., 2005), GI and progressive muscle relaxation were compared in regard to their effects in reducing in elderly cancer patients perioperative stress, which was expected to result in improving the patients' postoperative state, namely, analgesic requirement, pain perception, pulmonary function, duration of postoperative ileus, and fatigue after resection of colorectal cancer. Although patients in both groups evaluated positively the interventions, there were no effects in the postoperative analgesic consumption, subjective pain intensity at rest or while coughing, subjective fatigue evaluation, recovery of pulmonary function or duration of ileus.

In a second study (Stein et al., 2010) the effects of GI were compared with those of music therapy and standard care in patients scheduled to undergo coronary artery bypass graft. The interventions were administered by tapes preoperatively and intra-operatively. All patients completed questionnaires about the use of psychological and complementary medicine therapies, as well as other assessments preoperatively and at 1 week and 6 months postoperatively. No GI effects were detected postoperatively. In a third study (Danhauer et al., 2007) the effects of music or GI on reducing anxiety and perceived pain in colposcopy patients were compared with usual care. Patients in the three groups completed a questionnaire prior to the procedure and following it. There were no differences between the groups after the procedure in anxiety, pain or satisfaction with care, even in the case of patients who anticipated the most pain or scored high on anxiety prior to the procedure.

The following four studies report positive effects of GI in women with breast cancer undergoing chemotherapy. The participants in one study (Walker et al., 1999) were 96 women with newly diagnosed large or locally advanced breast cancer who got only standard care or in addition also relaxation and GI training. Tests for evaluating mood and quality of life were carried out before each of the six cycles of chemotherapy and 3 weeks after cycle 6, and clinical response to chemotherapy was evaluated by standard criteria after six cycles of chemotherapy. The intervention produced more relaxation, higher quality of life, and less emotional suppression. The two groups did not differ in clinical or pathological response to chemotherapy, but in the experimental group imagery vividness and degree of clinical response were positively correlated.

The participants in the second study were 66 patients with breast or gynecologic cancer undergoing brachytherapy (León-Pizarro et al., 2007). All patients received training for brachytherapy, but only those in the experimental group were trained in relaxation and GI. Questionnaires about anxiety, depression and quality of life were administered before, during and following brachytherapy. The findings showed a significant decrease in anxiety, depression and body discomfort in the experimental group.

In the third study the 60 participants were breast cancer patients undergoing chemotherapy, half of whom got training in progressive muscle relaxation and GI (Yoo et al., 2005). The results showed that the experimental group had less nausea and vomiting prior to the treatment and following it, as well as less anxiety, depression and hostility prior to each of six cycles of adjuvant chemotherapy, and higher quality of life scores 3 and 6 months after the treatment.

The effects that were assessed in the fourth study referred to pain, fatigue and sleep disturbances during treatment in advanced cancer patients with different diagnoses undergoing chemotherapy or radiotherapy (Kwekkeboom, Abbott-Anderson and Wanta, 2010). The intervention was in the form of tapes describing different strategies including GI, to which the patients could listen, as necessary, for symptom management for two weeks, keeping a log of symptom ratings with each use. Symptom scores at two weeks did not differ from baseline, but there were significant reductions in ratings of pain, fatigue, and sleep disturbance severity made immediately before and after use of the tapes.

GI effects in the treatment of pain. The use of GI for the treatment of pain appears to be quite common. Therefore, a special section is devoted to it although the theme could be presented also within the context of the preceding or following sections. The review by King (2010) on the application of GI to pain treatment deals only with cancer pain, which is itself a complex phenomenon due partly to the illness and partly to the treatments. King focused on studies performed from 2001 to 2008, which investigated the use of GI for relief of cancer pain. He found in the literature 5 studies which included pain as an outcome measure. Only in 2 studies the GI intervention resulted in a decrease of pain intensity and pain-related distress. In the first of these (Kwekkeboom, Kneip and Pearson, 2003) there were 62 hospitalized cancer patients who listened each one only once to a 12-minute tape of GI. Following this intervention there was a decrease of average pain intensity (on a numerical rating scale) in 90% of the participants. In the second study (Kwekkeboom, Wanta and Bumpus, 2008) there were 40 hospitalized cancer patients with pain who were administered over a 2-day period each two trials of an audiotaped intervention that consisted of the glove anesthesia of GI and progressive muscular relaxation. The results showed a decrease in pain intensity (on a numerical rating scale) in 31% and in pain-related distress in 37% in the experimental group as compared with decreases of 8% and 16% respectively, in the control group. The other 3 studies in King's review included 2 studies mentioned earlier (Haase et al., 2005; Leon-Pizzaro et al., 2007) and one (Anderson et al., 2006) in which 57cancer patients were administered a 20-minute audiotape which included positive mood statements and positive imagery suggestions. There was significant pain reduction immediately after listening to the tapes but after two weeks there were no effects in regard to pain, quality of life, mood, self efficacy or other symptoms.

Not surprisingly there are studies about the effect of GI on pain reduction also in regard to diagnoses other than cancer. One domain is musculoskeletal pain (Posadzki and Ernst, 2011). A search of six databases from their inception to May 2010 uncovered 9 studies reporting randomized controlled clinical trials in which GI was used as an intervention and pain as an outcome measure. In 8 of the 9 of studies the findings suggested that GI led to a significant reduction in pain.

Fibromyalgia is another domain in which pain alleviation by GI was tested. In one study 55 women with fibromyalgia were monitored for daily pain in a study with three groups: one received relaxation training and GI in "pleasant imagery", another received relaxation training and GI in "attention imagery" to the pain control systems, and a third was a simple control group (Fors, Sexton and Götestam, 2002). Significant differences were found in the pain-slopes between the three groups: the pleasant imagery but not the attention imagery group's slope declined significantly when compared with the control group. In another study (Menzies, Taylor and Bourguignon, 2006), 48 individuals with fibromyalgia were divided randomly into a standard care group and an experimental group whose members were given in addition a set of three audiotaped guided imagery scripts and were instructed to use at least one tape daily for 6 weeks and report weekly frequency of use. The results showed that GI did not affect pain (as measured by the McGill pain questionnaire) but brought about a decrease in the fibromyalgia impact and an increase in the ratings of self-efficacy for managing pain and other symptoms of fibromyalgia.

Osteoarthritis is a fourth illness in which the effects of GI on pain were studied. A search of the literature for studies of older adults (above 50) with chronic pain located 14 relevant studies. The review of these studies provided some support for the efficacy of progressive muscle relaxation plus GI for osteoarthritis pain (Monroe and Greco, 2007).

A longitudinal randomized assignment experimental design focused on studying the efficacy of GI and relaxation training for reducing pain, improving mobility, and reducing medication in older individuals with osteoarthris pain (Baird, Murawski and Wu, 2010). Thirty participants were randomly assigned to participate in the 4-month trial by using either

GI and relaxation or a sham intervention. The results showed that as compared to the control group, in the experimental group there was a significant reduction in pain from baseline to month 4, a significant improvement in mobility from baseline to month 2 and a reduction in the use of OTC and prescribed analgesic from baseline to month 4.

Also other types of pain react positively to GI intervention. In a study with women diagnosed with interstitial cystitis (IC) the experimental group listened twice daily for 8 weeks to a 25-minute GI compact disc which focused on healing the bladder, relaxing the pelvic-floor muscles, and quieting the nerves specifically involved in IC. Assessment questionnaires were administered at the beginning and end of the study including a visual analog scale for pain, a global response assessment, and 2-day voiding diaries. The results showed that 45% responded to GI. The responders had a significant improvement in pain scores at the end of the study if they also had at least a moderate improvement on the global response assessment (Carrico, Peters and Diokno, 2008).

Finally, it is notable that GI may affect positively pain also in children (Ball et al., 2003). Ten children with recurrent abdominal pain refractory to conventional treatment participated in the study. They were trained in relaxation and GI during 4 weekly 50-minute sessions. Pain diaries were completed at 0, 1, and 2 months. The results indicated that the children experienced a 67% decrease in pain during the therapy.

GI as a tool of healing physical disorders. There is some evidence that GI may facilitate the reduction of specific physical disorders. In one study with women diagnosed with uterine fibroids, several interventions that included also GI led to changes in fibroid size the sign (fibroids shrank or stopped growing in 22 patients in the experimental group compared with 3 in the control), reduction in bothersome symptoms, and higher patient satisfaction (Mehl-Madrona, 2002).

The above discussed study about the effects of GI on interstitial cystitis (Carrico et al., 2008) showed that the GI intervention affected not only the pain but also manifestations of the illness itself. As noted, the treatment group which listened twice daily for 8 weeks to a 25 minutes disk of GI focused on healing the bladder, relaxing the pelvic-floor muscles, and quieting the nerves involved in IC. About 45% responded to the GI. They had at least a moderate global response assessment, significant reductions in episodes of urgency and in the Interstitial Cystitis Symptom Index and Problem Index. These results suggest an impact of GI on symptoms of the disease.

Effects of GI on headaches were studied by comparing patients who listened to a GI tape with controls (Mannix et al., 1999). Those who listened to the GI tape improved in headache frequency, headache severity, patient global assessment, quality of life, and disability caused by headache. Further, of the GI patients than the controls reported that their headaches improved (21.7% vs 7.6) and they had significantly more improvement in three SF-36 domains: bodily pain, vitality and mental health. These results suggest that GI affects positively the management of chronic tension-type headache.

Spiegel and Moore (1997) analyzed the issue of whether GI and in particular the techniques involving the use of "positive mental images" of a strong army of white blood cells killing cancer cells have any impact on disease progression or survival in cancer. They concluded that there was no evidence to support claims of this kind. Despite claims to the contrary, no reliable evidence has shown that this technique affects disease progression or survival.

GI as a procedure for affecting immune system parameters. The effects of GI on the immune system have been studied quite extensively. The findings of these studies are of particular interest because failure of the proper functioning of the immune system may have deleterious effects on health.

On the basis of his review of studies done with healthy individuals or medical patients Trakhtenberg (2008) reached several conclusions. The more general ones were that GI and relaxation are related to the functioning of the immune system, and that interventions based on GI and relaxation may improve the functioning of the immune system by reducing stress, as noted above. The findings Trakhtenberg analyzed focused mainly on changes (increases or decreases) in the number of white blood cells (WBC) and changes in the nature of neutrophil adherence, which are related to changes in the functioning of the immune system. Studies show that an active cognitive act involved in the initial stages of GI is followed by decreases in neutrophil adherence while relaxation without an active imagery act is correlated with increases in neutrophil adherence (Hall et al., 1996). The mentioned decreases in WBC count occur only in the initial stages of enacting GI or relaxation exercises and the WBC tends to increase after 4-5 weeks of training (Donaldson, 2000; McGrady et al., 1992). The decreases in the initial stages of GI may be due to the stress of learning new GI techniques and focusing mentally on the images, whereas the increases in WBC count could result from enhanced relaxation (Donaldson, 2000). Another explanation is that the changes in the WBC count are not due to actual changes in the number of neutrophils but reflect merely changes in the movement of WBC and their locations in the body (Schneider et al., 1984; Achtenberg, 1985).

Another early study (Rider and Achtenberg, 1989) showed that cell-specific imagery may predict in which WBC category the changes will occur. Thus, neutrophils decreased significantly in the neutrophil imagery group, but lymphocytes did not. In the lymphocyte imagery group, only the lymphocyte count decreased. Similar findings supporting the importance of imagery specific for particular immune system parameters were reported in two studies with children. Olness et al. (1989) showed that sIgA levels increased significantly only in the group of children given a single session of self-hypnosis relaxation combined with specific suggestions about increasing immunoglobulins but remained unchanged in those given non-specific immune related suggestions, or a control group involved only in conversation. Similarly, in a study with 45 healthy children with recurrent upper respiratory tract infections there was an increase in concentration of sIgA and IgA/albumin ratio (a measure of local mucosal immunity) only with immune imagery (Hewson-Bower and Drummond, 1996).

We will mention next several studies targeting immune system parameters by means of GI interventions. Lehman et al. (2010) provided evidence in a randomized controlled trial that participation in a GI training produced decreases in serum IgE in adult patients with dust mite allergic asthma. The patients were treated over a 4-week period and assessed at baseline, after treatment and after 4 months for follow-up.

Rider et al. (1990) compared in healthy adults the effects of listening for 17 minutes to music inducing imagery or to the same music preceded by instructions and information about the immune system. Participants continued practicing on their own every other day for six weeks. sIgA was assessed at the beginning and end of the session before training, and at weeks, three and six. The results showed higher antibodies in both imagery groups, but sIgA was higher at weeks three and six only in the group with immune imagery. Salivary cortisol was the parameter assessed in a study with a training program of 13 weeks and 6 weeks follow-up (McKinney et al., 1997). Beneficial effects on cortisol were observed, but only in the follow-up assessment. Another study focused on the effects of relaxation and GI on the natural killer (NK) parameter (Zacharie et al., 1990). Ten healthy subjects were given for 10 days one 1-hour relaxation procedure and one combined relaxation and GI procedure, instructing them to imagine their immune system becoming very effective. There were no major changes in the composition of the major mononuclear leukocyte subsets but there was a significant increase in NK function. Similarly, 2 studies with early stage breast cancer patients assessed the immunological effects of hypnotic GI therapy and autogenic training. Both studies showed increased NK cell counts after 2 months of hypnosis treatment (Hudacek, 2007). Positive results were documented also in a further study with stage 1 breast cancer patients who were administered relaxation, GI, and biofeedback training. Significant effects were found in NK activity, mixed lymphocyte responsiveness (MLR), concanavalin A (Con-A) responsiveness, and the number of peripheral blood lymphocytes (PBL) (Gruber et al., 1993).

A further study with positive results was also done with breast cancer patients (in stages 0 to 2) (Lengacher et al., 2008). The experimental group got a relaxation and GI intervention and the control group got standard care. The effects of the intervention on immune function were measured by NK cell cytotoxicity and IL-2-activated NK cell activity prior to surgery and 4 weeks post-surgery. There were significant differences between the groups at 4 weeks post-surgery: NK cell cytotoxicity and IL-2 increased in the intervention group as compared to the control group.

Gruzelier et al. (2001a, 2001b) reported two studies with positive effects on immune parameters. The subjects were healthy medical students at exam times. In the first study a non-intervention control group was compared with a group receiving self-hypnosis instructions which included physical relaxation, immune imagery and cognitive alertness. In the second study subjects were allocated to immune imagery, or to relaxation imagery or to a control group. Immune parameters were obtained during the exams, and either four weeks before the exams (before training) or after the exams. The subjects practiced three times a week. The intervention buffered the effects of stress on immune functions in the students, and the comparison of self-hypnosis with and without immune imagery demonstrated positive effects following targeted imagery for immune function (especially in regard to NK CD4 and CD8) and also fewer winter viral infections. A third study (Gruzelier, 2002) showed in patients with virulent and chronic herpes simplex virus-2 (HSV-2) that six weeks of training almost halved recurrence, and upgraded immune functions, notably functional NK cell activity to HSV-1, as well as CD3, CD4, CD8 and CD16.

Probably the best randomized controlled study to date concerning effects of GI on immune parameters in breast cancer patients was done by Ermin et al. (2009). The participants were undergoing standard medical treatments. Those in the intervention group were taught relaxation and GI. Patients kept diaries of the frequency of relaxation practice and imagery vividness. On 10 occasions during the 37 weeks following the diagnosis, blood was taken for immunological assays CD phenotyping. In patients who got relaxation and GI the number of CD3+ (mature) T cells was significantly higher following chemotherapy and radiotherapy. Those who had high imagery ratingshad elevated levels of NK cell activity at the end of chemotherapy and at follow-up.

The next studies found no effects of GI on immune system parameters. Richardson et al. (1997) compared the effects of six weeks of imagery training on immune parameters in women who had completed treatment for primary breast cancer with the effects of standard care or social support. No results on the immune system were observed. Zacharie et al. (1994) measured cellular immune function on 3 investigation days 1 week apart in healthy subjects randomly selected for three groups: (1) a GI group instructed to enhance cellular immune function: (2) a relaxation group with no instructions about the immune system, and (3) a control group. In one study the assessed parameters were changes in monocyte chemotaxis (MC) and lymphocyte proliferative response (LPR) to three mitogens, while in another study NK cell activity was measured. The results show similar patterns of brief decreases in LPR and NK immediately after intervention on all investigation days in both intervention groups. Increases in MC were found in both intervention groups on day 1. On a follow-up investigation day in study 2, a brief stress task yielded a slight increase in NKCA. In study 2, the control group showed decreases in NK similar to those observed in the two intervention groups. In general, there were no significant changes in pre-intervention immune function throughout the investigation period.

Another study that reported inconsistent and nonsignificant results also focused on the parameter of NK number and cell activity in patients treated for Stage I or II breast cancer (Bakke, Purtzer and Newton, 2002). The intervention was a hypnotic-GI 8 weeks training and the assessments were made at baseline, after the training program and at the 3-month follow-up. The results showed an increase in absolute number of NK cells, but these were not maintained after the treatment ended at the 3-month follow-up.

GI from the Viewpoint of Clinical Practice

The review of studies done with GI demonstrates clearly some of the methodological shortcomings common in this domain of research. Two of the major issues are the absence of standardization in the performance of GI and the application of GI together with other affiliated methods, mainly relaxation and hypnosis. The present section will be devoted to describing a procedure of applying GI the author has been using extensively with cancer patients with different diagnoses in the framework of clinical practice. The procedure has been shaped with the intent of formalizing a module that is focused only on GI, is simple, easy to memorize, utilizes the sensory features of images, can be standardized, can be applied by patients on their own after a brief instruction and demonstration, and can be adjusted for different targets. The person who provides the guidance or instruction in GI is referred to as therapist or guided-imagery instructor.

Description of the Kreitler procedure for guided imagery: There are four main stages in the training of the Kreitler procedure for GI.

Stage 1: The first stage is designed to introduce the participant to the procedure in general terms. The major points made in introducing the procedure are the following:

1. The procedure is designed to enable a person to give himself/herself orders or instructions with a good chance that they are fulfilled if the procedure is implemented correctly.

2. The orders or instructions one can give oneself may refer to different domains but the major purpose in training in the present context is limited to physical health issues.

3. Success in implementing the procedure does not require believing in anything, only enacting the procedure according to the guidelines.

4. The procedure is designed to be implemented by the person himself/herself without the intervention of others.

5. The procedure may be enacted repeatedly, in regard to the same goal, with or without variations in the adequate components ("the substance", see Stage 2, #1). There is a good chance that attaining the goals set for the procedure may be promoted and made easier the more the procedure is enacted.

6. The same procedure may be enacted by the individual in regard to different goals, although each time it is enacted there should be only one goal.

7. The procedure is guided imagery and not hypnosis, although some people may call it hypnosis or self- hypnosis.

8. The major point is to learn to implement the procedure correctly.

Stage 2: The second stage is designed to describe to the participant the major components and structure of the procedure. The main points are the following:

1. Guided imagery consists of two components, which may be called "the frame" and "the substance".

2. "The frame" is fixed and should not be changed (without a good reason), because it functions as a kind of code facilitating the entrance into the state adequate for guided imagery. The contents and the structure of "the frame" express clearly the notion that guided imagery depends totally on the participant and his/her decisions and remains all the time under one's control. "The frame" consists of two arms: the arm of the entrance and the arm of the exit.

   The arm of the entrance of "the frame" is defined by three items: (a) the decision to perform guided imagery, i.e., to enter the state of mind adequate for enacting guided imagery; (b) selecting a specific personal number (any number from 6 to 12) and counting the number of one's breaths in accordance with this number (the breaths need not be of any specific nature in terms of speed, or depth, just "natural" and their character may change from one act of guided imagery to another); and (c) selecting a certain image that one enacts while entering the state of mind adequate for guided imagery, for example, entering a certain place, going down the stairs, climbing up the stairs, entering a garden, going to the mall etc. It is emphasized that this image should not be changed from one act of guided imagery to another, and especially that the image has nothing to do with the goal of the particular act of guided imagery that one has selected or decided upon.

   The arm of the exit of "the frame" consists of components similar to those that define the entrance arm, but in reverse form. Thus, the first component is the decision to get out of the state of mind adequate for enacting guided imagery; the second component is counting the set number of breaths in reverse order, i.e., if in the entrance arm one counted from 1 to say 7, then in the exit arm one is instructed to count the breaths in the reverse order: 7, 6, 5 etc. up to 1 and zero that marks the end;

the third component is an image whereby the participant reverses the act of the entrance arm, e.g., exits the place he or she entered in the entrance arm or if one went down the stairs then going up, etc. Thus, the entrance and the exit arms are the reverse of each other. The whole procedure is concluded with a light opening and closing of the fists twice which marks symbolically the end of the guided imagery act.

3. "The substance" is the major phase of the whole procedure, actually the reason why the guided imagery is enacted. It refers to a particular issue or target, which is determined ahead of time, for example, relaxation, speeding up the healing of a wound, diminishing a certain pain, or promoting the production of neutrophils or platelets. The five following points are presented as defining the manner in which "the substance" should be performed:

(a) The goal and the given orders should be expressed only in the form of images. The images may refer to any of the senses. Examples and training are provided for translating goals into images (see stage 3);

(b) The goal should be specific as far as possible, i.e., specific in regard to the target (e.g., neutrophils, or platelets, or the pain in the knee), in regard to the range or scope (e.g., some of the pain should be alleviated), and even in regard to the time frame (e.g., the specified target should be attained until a particular time). Specificity also means that when dealing for example with a physiological symptom, the focus should be exclusively on that symptom and not on any other accompanying or affiliated reactions (e.g., when focusing on alleviating pain it is suggested that the accompanying distress be overlooked in the course of the specific guided imagery act, although it can be the focus of another guided imagery act). Specificity further implies that no two goals are to be handled in the framework of the same guided imagery act.

(c) The goal and the orders should be phrased in a syntactically positive or active form. For example in regard to pain, the order should not be that the pain is no longer there but rather that it was packed and thrown away, or that it dissipates or evaporates or is crushed in some form; in regard to a tumor, the goal and the orders should not be that there is no tumor any more but that it is cut or pulverized or dehydrated etc. The emphasis in "positive" is on the form of expression and not on positive thinking, as some people may tend to understand this phrase.

(d) The goal and the orders should be physiologically adequate as far as possible. This factor relates specifically to applications in the health domain. In other domains this factor signifies "operational adequacy" which indicates that the designed act can be performed in reality. Physiological adequacy implies that the act is envisaged in terms that approximate as much as possible the actual physiological operation. For example, in regard to nausea, GI may refer to the physiological processes involved in the production of nausea in the brain or in the gastrointestinal tract; in regard to neutrophil increases, the GI act may refer to the actual production of neutrophils in the bone marrow, including the existing information about the form and behavior of the neutrophils.

Physiological adequacy also means that GI should not be enacted in regard to processes that may possibly be obstructed, for example, no instructions for urine flow through the urinary tract should be given when the urinary tract is obstructed for example by a tumor.

Another limitation on the factor of physiological adequacy is personal attitudes and the cognitive state of the individual. Young children may find it difficult to understand or focus on actual physiological processes. The same may hold for elderly patients. Personal attitudes of denial or unwillingness to confront the physiological problem may limit the individual's readiness to focus on a physiologically coherent image and prefer instead a metaphorical one.

(e) The goal and the orders should be psychologically adequate for the individual. This means that the images involved in the guided imagery act should be made to conform to the individual's tendencies, and preferably be shaped by the individual. If the images are suggested by the therapist or guided-imagery instructor, it is advisable to check whether the images do not evoke rejection, anxiety or unpleasantness in the subject. For example, when relaxation is the goal, an image such as "lying on the beach" should not be used without checking beforehand whether the individual does not reject the beach scene with the sun, the noise and the sand. Again, when diminishing a tumor is the goal, it would be advisable to check whether the patient is at all ready or willing to imagine the tumor.

4. "A guided imagery act" includes an entrance arm, the substance in regard to some target, sometimes the post-imagery order, the exit arm, and opening and closing the fists twice. The post-imagery order is an optional component of the guided imagery act. It refers to instructions given in regard to continuation of the goal attainment also in the course of the period between one guided imagery act and another (e.g., "I rely on you neutrophils to go on increasing also while I get out of the guided imagery state") or sometimes in regard to the next guided imagery act (e.g., "I expect to be able to attain the same or an even better state of relaxation next time I perform guided imagery for relaxation").

Stage 3: The third stage is designed to elaborate and train the image component of guided imagery. The major points are the following:

a. Images may be of different sensory domains. It is necessary to find out which are the favored images by the individual. Most people prefer the visual or auditory images. An individual should be encouraged to use the kind of image with which he/she is most familiar or comfortable. However, it is possible or even desirable to elaborate images through the use of multiple sensory-based images. Thus, even if the major image is visual, it may be further elaborated or amplified in terms of auditory, olfactory and tactile images.

b. Thinking in terms of images is promoted by focusing on the images and avoiding the use of words during the guided imagery act. Words may inhibit the use of images especially in individuals who are not particularly adept at thinking in terms of images. Closing one's eyes during the guided imagery act is another advice that holds mainly for those who are inexperienced in regard to images or in the first phases of performing guided imagery acts. The reason is that perceptual images may gain preference over internally-produced images in individuals who are relatively inexperienced in regard to images.

c. The individual may be involved in the production of images in different degrees. The least involvement is represented by adopting or relying on an image suggested by the therapist or guided magery instructor. There is some involvement even in this case because the individual is required to reproduce the suggested image for himself or herself. A higher degree of involvement is required when the image suggested by the therapist or guided magery instructor is incomplete. The suggested image is merely a frame and needs to be elaborated and implemented by the individual. For example, the image suggested for pain may be "a color" without indicating which color and what happens to the color in the course of the guided imagery act (e.g., whether it fades away, is blurred, is darkened, is covered or obliterated by another color, is washed away, etc.). Sometimes an image suggested by the therapist is amended by the individual, for example, if the suggested image is a hand or glove that absorbs tensions and pain, the individual may feel threatened by the hand image and may replace it by a flower or handkerchief or shawl that suck the tension and pain. The highest degree of involvement is presented by the case when the individual produces the image by himself/herself with or without some guidance from the therapist. This mostly takes place prior to the enactment of the guided imagery act although the image may be further elaborated in the course of the guided imagery itself.

d. Images may have different degrees of concreteness and controllability. For guided imagery it is advisable to use images that are maximally concrete, namely, endowed with sensory or perceptual characteristics, and under the control of the individual, namely, may be changed or shaped in line with the targets of the guided imagery.

Individuals are mostly unaware to which degree their images are concrete or controllable by them. In order to promote awareness of the character of images, a brief exercise is enacted with the patients. They are requested to close their eyes and imagine for example a cat. The exercise has two phases administered in one sequence. In the first phase the therapist asks questions, such as "Does the cat have a tail? Can you see the hairs in the ears of the cat? Are the cat's eyes open or closed? Can you see the cat's whiskers which are long and far apart? " The second phase starts with the statement "Let's get the cat to move". The therapist proceeds with instructions, such as "the cat starts walking slowly; now the cat speeds up a little; the cat stops and raises its head, it apparently heard some bird twittering up in the branches of a tree; the cat stops by a fence, measures the height and… jumps on the fence; let's leave it there thinking of the bird for lunch". The patient is asked to answer the questions only after the imagery exercise. The answers to the questions of the first phase show the degree to which the patient's image was concrete. The image lacks concreteness if the patient answers that at least some of the features became apparent only after the therapist asked the question (e.g., "I saw the whiskers only after you asked"). This experience helps the patient to become aware of what a concrete image means. The answers of the patient in regard to the second phase of the exercise serve to check to what degree the patient has control over his/her images. The control over the imagery is incomplete if the patient answers that at least in some cases the cat did not 'perform' the actions suggested by the therapist (e.g., it did not raise its head).

When the images are not optimally concrete or controllable, the patient is advised to perform some training for improving these properties. Concreteness is trained by applying Pylyshyn's (1999) notion of the cognitive penetrability of images. The patient is instructed to close one's eyes and form an image of a common object available in the immediate surroundings, e.g., a cup. The next instruction is to open one's eyes, notice any feature in the cup that was not represented in one's image of the cup and insert it in the image. This instruction is repeated in regard to another feature. The patient is advised to train this procedure in regard to different objects, without necessarily elaborating optimally any of the images. Controlling images is trained by imagining some object, say a leaf in midair which is being moved by a very weak air current, or a bud of a flower whose petals open very slowly. It is emphasized to the patient that both kinds of exercises may be done just for a few seconds, for several days. They are expected to be helpful because most people dispose over the capacity for imagery but many have not used it a lot in adulthood. Hence, the exercises are actually designed more to refresh the function of imagery rather than to train it.

e. Evoking in the patient the personal-subjective mode of meanings is another possible means of enhancing the imagery component and the effectiveness of the guided imagery act. This means is merely optional and is probably involved to some degree by the mere evocation of images, because images are the preferred means of expression of personal meanings (Kreitler, 2009, 2012).

The personal-subjective mode of meanings has been developed and studied in the framework of the Kreitler theory of meaning (Kreitler,1965, 1999, 2001, 2002; Kreitler and Kreitler, 1972, 1990). It will be described briefly in this context.

The personal-subjective mode of meaning is one of two forms in which meanings are expressed. The first is the interpersonally-shared mode of meaning which is applied mainly for expressing and communicating lexically defined and commonly used meanings. It is characterized by the attributive and comparative types of relation which describe the form in which the theme or referent is related to the contents that is used to describe it. Thus, the attributive type of relation relates the contents to the referent directly in terms of agent to qualities (e.g., Flower - in the garden) or agent to action (e.g., Lion - can roar). The comparative type of relation relates the contents to the referent through the mediation of another referent on the same level of abstractness, in one of the following forms by way of similarity (e.g., Sea - has the same color as the sky), difference (e.g., House - unlike a tent is built of wood or bricks), complementarity (e.g., Wife - has a husband and husband has a wife), and relationality (e.g., Highway - broader than a path).

The personal-subjective mode of meaning is applied mainly for expressing and communicating personal meanings. It is characterized by the exemplifying-illustrative and the metaphoric-symbolic types of relation which describe particular forms of relating contents to a referent.

The exemplifying-illustrative type of relation relates the contents to the referent by way of an example, in the form of an instance (e.g., Wisdom - Moses), an image portraying a situation (e.g., Motherhood - A woman holding a baby in her arms) or a scene with dynamic elements (e.g., Aggression - An unemployed person comes to the government agency for employment, the clerk tells him that there is no work for him, the person feels warm anger rising in him, his fists clench, his vision becomes blurred etc.).

The metaphoric-symbolic type of relation relates the contents to the referent in a mediated way using contents which is not conventionally related to the referent, in the form of an interpretation (e.g., Life - the unknown known), metaphor (an image related interpretatively to a more abstract referent, e.g., Wisdom - cool water in the desert at noon), or symbol (a metaphoric image that resolves contrasting elements, e.g., Love - a fire that produces and consumes).

Studies have shown that inducing the personal-subjective mode of meaning in individuals by cognitively-based psychological means produces marked changes in cognitive functioning, which include mainly thinking in terms of images, handling images in better ways, improved visual memory, enhanced intuition, comprehending and constructing metaphors, and so on (Kreitler, 2009, 2011). Of particular importance is the finding that induction of the personal-subjective mode of meaning enhances the availability and accessibility of information about oneself including one's physical and physiological state (Kreitler, 2012).

The induction of the personal-subjective mode of meaning is based on directed meaning elaboration. It is done by requesting the participant to express meanings of common words in terms of the described forms of relation, namely, by providing examples or exemplifying situations or scenes, metaphors or symbols. The induction may be done verbally in a session with a therapist or through materials on the internet (Rotstein, Maimon and Kreitler, 2012). The induction is continued until the majority of meaning expressions provided by the participant conform to the requested mode of meaning, namely, they are examples or metaphors. When the goal of the induction is to produce a preparatory state of mind for the guided image procedure, a brief induction that lasts no longer than 5-8 minutes may suffice.

Stage 4: The fourth stage is designed to put the whole procedure together so that it becomes available to the patient. This is done primarily by enacting the procedure with the patient from beginning to end in regard to a goal, such as relaxation. The enactment is brief and does not last more than 5 minutes. After its completion the patient is interviewed about his or her feelings and the total experience. The different aspects are explained and discussed with the patient.

The procedure may be enacted together with the patient as many times as necessary until the patient may feel confident enough to proceed on one's own. The enactment of the patient on one's own is limited to targets that have been defined and clarified together with the therapist. Further meetings may be necessary for keeping track of implementation by the patient and resolving problems that may be encountered. If the patient desires or feels it necessary, the guided imagery acts are extended to targets beyond those that have been originally defined and practiced.

*Advantages and risks of GI.*The major advantage of GI is that it often produces beneficial results for the patients in the medical context. An additional advantage is that it is often accompanied by increased self confidence and sense of control emanating from the fact that the patient feels empowered. These beneficial effects depend on performing GI in a correct manner following precisely the guidelines. However, often the instructors in GI are not professionals who understand the procedure in a manner that enables them to guide the patients in an optimal and adequate way. Another risk is that some patients may decide to rely for recovery exclusively on GI without applying the standard medical treatments. Both kinds of risks are shared by GI with other complementary therapeutic procedures and both risks may be moderated or avoided when GI is applied mainly by professional instructors.

REFERENCES

Achterberg, J. (1985). Imagery in healing. Boston, MA: Shambala.

Anderson, K., Cohen, M., Mendoza, T., Guo, H., Harle, M., and Cleeland, C. (2006). Brief cognitive-behavioral audiotape interventions for cancer-related pain. *Cancer*, 107, 207-214.

Antonietti, A., and Colombo, B. (2011). Mental imagery as a strategy to enhance creativity in children. *Imagination, Cognition and Personality*, 31, 63-77.

Baird, C. L., Murawski, M. M., and Wu, J. (2010). Efficacy of guided imagery with relaxation for osteoarthritis symptoms and medication intake. *Pain Management Nursing*, 11, 56-65.

Bakke, A.C., Purtzer, M.Z., and Newton, P. (2002). The effect of hypnotic- guided imagery on psychological well-being and immune function in patients with prior breast cancer. *Journal of Psychosomatic Research*, 53, 1131-1137.

Ball, T.M., Shapiro, D.E., Monheim, C.J., and Weydert, J.A. (2003). A pilot study of the use of guided imagery for the treatment of recurrent abdominal pain in children. *Clinical Pediatrics*, 42, 527-532.

Ben-Arye, E., Karkabi, S., Shapira, C., Schiff, E., Lavie, O., and Keshet, Y. (2009). Complementary medicine in the primary care setting: Results of a survey of gender and cultural patterns in Israel. *Gender Medicine*, 6, 384-397.

Bensafi, M., Porter, J., Pouliot, S., Mainland, J., Johnson, B., Zelano, C., Young, N., Bremner, E., Aframian, D., Khan, R., and Sobel, N. (2003) Olfactomotor activity during imagery mimics that during perception. *Nature Neuroscience*, 6, 1142–1144.

Berg, C.J., Snyder, C.R., and Hamilton, N. (2008). The effectiveness of a hope intervention in coping with cold pressor pain. *Journal of Health Psychology*, 13, 804-809.

Brewin, C.R., Dalgleish, T., Joseph, S.A. (1996). A dual representation-theory of posttraumatic-stress-disorder. *Psychological Review*, 103, 670-686.

Broadbent, E., Kahokehr, A., Booth, R.J., Thomas, J., Windsor, J.A., Buchanan, C.M., Wheeler, B.R., Sammour, T., and Hill, A.G. (2012). A brief relaxation intervention reduces stress and improves surgical wound healing response: a randomised trial. *Brain, Behavior, and Immunity*, 26, 212-217.

Carrico, D. J., Peters, K. M., and Diokno, A. C. (2008). Guided imagery for women with interstitial cystitis: results of a prospective, randomized controlled pilot study. *Journal of Alternative and Complementary Medicine*, 14, 53-60.

Clark, C. D. (1998). Childhood imagination in the face of chronic illness. In T.R. Sarbin, J. de Rivera, J. (Eds.), (1998). Believed-in imaginings: The narrative construction of reality (pp. 87-100). Washington, DC, US: American Psychological Association.

Clement, J. (2008). Creative model construction in scientists and students: The role of imagery, analogy, and mental simulation. Dordrecht, The Netherlands: Springer.

Cotton, S., Luberto, C.M., Yi, M.S., and Tsevat, J. (2011). Complementary and alternative medicine behaviors and beliefs in urban adolescents with asthma. *The Journal of Asthma*, 48, 531-538.

Danhauer, S.C., Marler, B., Rutherford, C.A., Lovato, J.F., Asbury, D.Y., McQuellon, R.P., and Miller, B.E. (2007). Music or guided imagery for women undergoing colposcopy: a randomized controlled study of effects on anxiety, perceived pain, and patient satisfaction. *Journal of Lower Genital Tract Diseases*, 11, 39-45.

Donaldson, V. W. (2000). A clinical study of visualization on depressed white blood cell count in medical patients. *Applied Psychophysiology and Biofeedback*, 25, 230–235.

Eremin, O., Walker, M.B., Simpson, .E, Heys, S.D., Ah-See, A.K., Hutcheon, A.W., Ogston, K.N., Sarkar, T.K., Segar, A., and Walker, L.G. (2009). Immuno-modulatory effects of relaxation training and GI in women with locally advanced breast cancer undergoing multimodality therapy: a randomised controlled trial. *Breast*, 18, 17-25.

Foote, W.W. (1996). Guided-imagery therapy. In B.W. Scotton, A. B. Chinen, and J. R. Battista (Eds.), Textbook of transpersonal psychiatry and psychology (pp. 355–365). New York: Basic Books.

Fors, E.A., Sexton, H., and Götestam, K.G. (2002). The effect of GI and amitriptyline on daily fibromyalgia pain: a prospective, randomized, controlled trial. *Journal of Psychiatric Research*, 36, 179-187.

Fouladbakhsh, J. M., and Stommel, M. (2010). Gender, symptom experience, and use of complementary and alternative medicine practices among cancer survivors in the U.S. cancer population. *Oncology Nursing Forum*, 37, E7-E15.

Frankl, V. E. (1959). Man's search for meaning. Boston, MA: Beacon Press.

Gafner, G. (2010). Techniques of hypnotic induction. Bethel, CT: Crown House Publishing. Gary, C. W. (2011). Hypnotically enhanced interactive cognitive rehearsal. In Rosenthal, H. G. (Ed.), Favorite counseling and therapy techniques (2nd ed.), (pp. 81-84). New York, NY, US: Routledge/Taylor and Francis Group.

Gordon, J.S., Staples, J.K., Blyta, A., Bytyqi, M., and Wilson, A.T. (2008). Treatment of posttraumatic stress disorder in postwar Kosovar adolescents using mind-body skills groups: a randomized controlled trial. *The Journal of Clinical Psychiatry*, 69, 1469-1476.

Goldstein, A.B., and Russ, S.W. (2000–2001). Understanding children's literature and its relationship to fantasy ability and coping. *Imagination, Cognition, and Personality*, 20, 105-126.

Gruber, B.L., Hersh, S.P., Hall, N.R., Waletzky, L.R., Kunz, J.F., Carpenter, J.K., Kverno, K.S., and Weiss, S.M. (1993). Immunological responses of breast cancer patients to behavioral interventions. *Biofeedback and Self-Regulation*, 18, 1-22.

Gruzelier, J.H., Smith, F., Nagy, A., and Henderson, D. (2001a). Cellular and humoral immunity, mood and exam stress: the influences of self hypnosis and personality predictors. *International Journal of Psychophysiology*, 41, 55–71.

Gruzelier, J.H., Levy, J.,Williams, J.D., and Henderson, D. (2001b). Selfhypnosis and exam stress: comparing immune and relaxation-related imagery for influences on immunity, health and mood. *Contemporary Hypnosis*, 18, 97-110.

Gruzelier, J. H. (2002). A review of the impact of hypnosis, relaxation, guided imagery and individual differences on aspects of immunity and health. *Stress*, 5, 147-163.

Gyselinck, V., and Pazzaglia, F. (Eds.) (2012). From mental imagery to spatial cognition an language: Essays in honor of Michel Denis. London, UK: Psychology Press [Psychology Press Festschrift Series].

Gary, C. W. (2011). Hypnotically enhanced interactive cognitive rehearsal. In Rosenthal, H. G. (Ed.), Favorite counseling and therapy techniques (2nd ed.), (pp. 81-84). New York, NY, US: Routledge/Taylor and Francis Group.

Haase, O., Schwenk, W., Hermann, C., and Miller, J. M. (2005). Guided imagery and relaxation in conventional colorectal resections: a randomized, controlled, partially blinded trial. *Diseases of the Colon and Rectum*, 48, 1955-1963.

Hall, H. R., Papas, A., Tosi, M., and Olness, K. (1996). Directional changes in neutrophiladherence following passive resting versus active imagery. *International Journal of Neuroscience*, 85, 185–194.

Heinschel, J. A. (2002). A descriptive study of the interactive guided imagery experience. *Journal of Holistic Nursing*, 20, 325–346.

Hewson-Bower, B.,and Drummond, P.D. (1996). Secretory immunoglobulin A increases during relaxation in children with and without recurrent upper respiratory tract infections. *Journal of Developmental and Behavioral Pediatrics,* 17, 311–316.

Hilgard, E. (1977). Divided consciousnesss: Multiple controls in humn thought and action. New York: Wiley and Sons.

Hudacek, K. D. (2007). A review of the effects of hypnosis on the immune system in breast cancer patients: a brief communication. *The International Journal of Clinical and Experimental Hypnosis*, 55, 411-425.

Jeannerod, M. (1994). The representing brain: Neural correlates of motor intention and imagery. *Behavioral and Brain Sciences*, 17, 187-245.

Jing, X., Wu, P., Liu, F., Wu, B., and Miao, D. (2011). Guided imagery, anxiety, heart rate, and heart rate variability during centrifuge training. *Aviation, Space, and Environmental Medicine*, 82, 92-96.

Kabat-Zinn, J. (1990). *Full catastrophe living*. New York: Delta Books.

Kozak, L.E., Kayes, L., McCarty, R., Walkinshaw, C., Congdon, S., Kleinberger, J., Hartman, V., and Standish, L.J. (2008-2009). Use of complementary and alternative medicine (CAM) by Washington State hospices. *The American Journal of Hospice and Palliative Care*, 25,463-468.

Kemper, K.J., and Wornham, W.L. (2001). Consultations for holistic pediatric services for inpatients and outpatient oncology patients at a children's hospital. *Archives of Pediatrics and Adolescent Medicine*, 155, 449-454.

King, K. (2010). A review of the effects of guided imagery on cancer patients with pain. *Complementary Health Practice Review*, 15, 98-107.

Klatzky, R. L., Lederman, S. J., and Matula, D. E. (1991). Imagined haptic exploration in judgments of object properties. *Journal of experimental psychology. Learning, memory, and cognition*, 17, 314-322.

Kosslyn, S. (1994). Image and brain: The resolution of the imagery debate. Cambridge, MA: MIT Press.

Kreitler, S. (1965). Symbolschöpfung und Symbolerfassung: Eine Experimentalpsychologische Studie (The formation and perception of symbols: Experimental studies). Munich-Basel: Reinhardt Verlag.

Kreitler, S. (1999). Consciousness and meaning. In J. Singer and P. Salovey (Eds.), At play in the fields of consciousness: Essays in honor of Jerome L. Singer (pp. 175-206). Mahwah, NJ: Erlbaum.

Kreitler, S. (2001). Psychological perspective on virtual reality. In A. Riegel, M. F. Peschl, K. Edlinger, G. Fleck and W. Feigl (Eds.), Virtual reality: Cognitive foundations, technological issues and philosophical implications (pp. 33-44). Frankfurt, Germany: Peter Lang.

Kreitler, S. (2002). Consciousness and states of consciousness: An evolutionary perspective. *Evolution and Cognition*, 8, 27-42.

Kreitler, S. (2009). Altered states of consciousness as structural variations of the cognitive system. In E. Franco (Ed., in collab. with D. Eigner), Yogic perception, meditation and altered states of consciousness (pp. 407-434). Vienna, Austria: Oestrreichische Akademie der Wissenschaften.

Kreitler, S. (2011). The psychosemantic approach to logic. In S. Kreitler, L. Ropolyi, D. Eigner and G. Fleck (Eds.) Systems of logic and the construction of order (pp. 33-60). Bern, New York, Vienna: Peter Lang.

Kreitler, S. (2012). Consciousness and knowledge: The psychosemantic approach. In S. Kreitler and O. Maimon (Eds.), Consciousness: Its nature and functions (chp.13). Hauppauge, NY: Nova Publishers.

Kreitler, H., and Kreitler, S. (1972). Psychology of the arts. Durham, NC: Duke University Press.

Kreitler, S., and Kreitler, H. (1990). The cognitive foundations of personality traits. New York: Plenum.

Kwekkeboom, K., Kneip, J., and Pearson, L. (2003). A pilot study to predict success with guided imagery for cancer pain. *Pain Management Nursing*, 4, 112-123.

Kwekkeboom, K., Wanta, B., and Bumpus, M. (2008). Individual difference variables and the effects of progressive muscle relaxation and analgesic imagery interventions on cancer pain. *Journal of Pain and Symptom Management*, 36, 604-615.

Kwekkeboom, K.L., Abbott-Anderson, K., and Wanta, B. (2010). Feasibility of a patient-controlled cognitive-behavioral intervention for pain, fatigue, and sleep disturbance in cancer. *Oncology Nursing Forum*, 37, E151-E159.

Lahmann, C., Henningsen, P., Schulz, C., Schuster, T., Sauer, N., Noll-Hussong, M., Ronel, J., Tritt, K., and Loew, T. (2010). Effects of functional relaxation and guided imagery on IgE in dust-mite allergic adult asthmatics: a randomized, controlled clinical trial. *The Journal of Nervous and Mental Disease*, 198, 125-130.

Lambert, S. A. (1996). The effects of hypnosis/ guided imagery on the postoperative course of children. *Journal of Developmental and Behavioral Pediatrics*, 17, 307-310.

Lee, S.-H., Kravitz, D. J., and Baker, C. I. (2012). Disentangling visual imagery and perception of real-world objects. *NeuroImage*, 59, 4064-4073.

Lengacher, C.A., Bennett, M.P., Gonzalez, L., Gilvary, D., Cox, C.E., Cantor, A., Jacobsen, P.B., Yang, C., and Djeu, J. (2008). Immune responses to guided imagery during breast cancer treatment. *Biological Research for Nursing*, 9, 205-214.

León-Pizarro, C., Gich, I., Barthe, E., Rovirosa, A., Farrús, B., Casas, F., Verger, E., Biete, A., Craven-Bartle, J., Sierra, J., and Arcusa A. (2007). A randomized trial of the effect of training in relaxation and guided imagery techniques in improving psychological and quality-of-life indices for gynecologic and breast brachytherapy patients. *Psycho-Oncology*, 16, 971-979.

Lin, Y.C., Lee, A.C., Kemper, K.J., and Berde, C.B. (2005). Use of complementary and alternative medicine in pediatric pain management service: a survey. *Pain Medicine*, 6, 452-558.

Lynn, S.J., Pintar, J. and Rhue, J.W. (1997). Fantasy proneness, dissociation, and narrative construction. In S. Krippner and S. M. Powers (Eds.), Broken images broken selves: dissociative narratives in clinical practice (pp. 274-304). Washington: Bruner-Mazel Publishers.

Mannix, L.K., Chandurkar, R.S., Rybicki, L.A., Tusek, D.L.., and Solomon, G. D. (1999). Effect of guided imagery on quality of life for patients with chronic tension-type headache. *Headache*, 39, 326-334.

Mattie, P., and Munroe-Chandler, K. (2012). Examining the relationship between mental toughness and imagery use. *Journal of Applied Sport Psychology*, 24, 144-156.

Mannix, L.K., Chandurkar, R.S., Rybicki, L.A., Tusek, D.L.., and Solomon, G. D. (1999). Effect of guided imagery on quality of life for patients with chronic tension-type headache. *Headache*, 39, 326-334.

McGrady, A., Conrad, P., Dickey, D., Garman, D., Farris, E., and Schumann-Brzezinski, C. (1992). The effects of biofeedback-assisted relaxation on cell-mediated immunity, cortisol, and white blood cell count in healthy adult subjects. *Journal of Behavioral Medicine*, 15, 343–354.

Mehl-Madrona, L. (2002). Complementary medicine treatment of uterine fibroids: a pilot study. *Alternative Therapies in Health and Medicine*, 8, 34-36, 38-40, 42, 44-46.

Menzies, V., Taylor, A.G.., and Bourguignon, C. (2006). Effects of guided imagery on outcomes of pain, functional status, and self-efficacy in persons diagnosed with fibromyalgia. *Journal of Alternative and Complementary Medicine*, 12, 23-30.

Moore, K. C., and Carlson, M. P. (2012). Students' images of problem contexts when solving applied problems. *Journal of Mathematical Behavior*, 31, 48-59.

Moreau, D., Mansy-Dannay, A., Clerc, J., and Guerrién, A. (2011). Spatial ability and motor performance: Assessing mental rotation processes in elite and novice athletes. *International Journal of Sport Psychology*, 42, 525-547.

Morone, N. E., and Greco, C. M. (2007). Mind-body interventions for chronic pain in older adults: a structured review. *Pain Medicine*, 8, 359-375.

Newton, N. (1993). The sensorimotor theory of cognition. *Pragmatics and Cognition*, 1, 267-305.

Newton, N. (1982). Experience and imagery. *Southern Journal of Philosophy*, 20, 475–487.

Olness, K., Culbert, T. and Den, D. (1989). Self-regulation of salivary immunoglobulin A by children. *Pediatrics*, 83, 66–71.

O'Donnell, J. J., Maurice, S. C., and Beattie, T. F. (2002). Emergency analgesia in the paediatric population: Part III non-pharmacological measures of pain relief and anxiolysis. *Emergency Medicine Journal*, 19, 195–197.

Paige, M., and Munroe-Chandler, K. (2012). Examining the relationship between mental toughness and imagery use. *Journal of Applied Sport Psychology*, 24, 144-156.

Paivio , A. (1971). Imagery and verbal processes. New York: Holt, Rinehart, and Winston. (Reprinted 1979, Hillsdale, NJ: Lawrence Erlbaum Associates).

Palmiero, M., Cardi, V., and Belardinelli, M. O. (2011). The role of vividness of visual mental imagery on different dimensions of creativity. *Creativity Research Journal*, 23, 372-375.

Pearlman, M. Y., Schwalbe, K. A., and Cloltre, M. (2010). Coping skills for grieving children. In Pearlman, M. Y., Schwalbe, K. A., and Cloltre, M. (Eds.), *Grief in childhood: Fundamentals of treatment in clinical practice* (pp. 165-181). Washington, DC, US: American Psychological Association.

Posadzki, P., and Enst, E. (2011). Guided imagery for musculoskeletal pain: a systematic review. *The Clinical Journal of Pain*, 27, 648-53.

Puchalski, L. (2000). The use of alternative and complementary medicine in radiology today. *Radiology Management*, 22, 51-55.

Pylyshyn, Z. (1999). Is vision continuous with cognition? The case of impenetrability of visual perception. *Behavioral and Brain Sciences*, 22, 341–423.

Reisberg, D. (Ed.) (1992). Auditory imagery. Hillsdale, NJ: Erlbaum. Richardson, M.A., Post-White, J., Grimm, E.A., Moye, L.A., Singletary, S.A., and Justice, B. (1997). Coping, life attitudes, and immune responses to imagery and group support after breast cancer treatment. *Alternative Therapy*, 3, 62–70.

Rider, M.S., Achterberg, J., Lawlis, G.F., Goven, A., Toledo, R., and Butler, J.R. (1990). Effect of immune system imagery on secretory IgA. *Biofeedback Self-regulation*, 15, 317–323.

Rider, M.S., Floyd, J.W., and Kirkpatrick, J. (1985). The effect of music, therapy, and relaxation on adrenal corticosteroids and the re-entrainment of circadian rhythms. *Journal of Music Therapy*, 22, 46-58.

Rider, M. S., and Achterberg, J. (1989). Effect of music-assisted imagery on neutrophils and lymphocytes. *Biofeedback and Self-regulation*, 14, 247–257.

Roeckelein, J. E. (2004). Imagery in psychology: A reference guide. Westport, CT: Greenwood Publishing Group.

Rossman, M. L. (2002). Interactive guided imagery as a way to access patient strengths during cancer treatment. *Integrative Cancer Therapies*, 1, 162-165.

Rotstein, Y., Maimon, O., and Kreitler, S. (2012). Cognitive effects of states of consciousness: Do changes in states of consciousness affect judgments and evaluations? In S. Kreitler, and O. Maimon (Eds.), *Consciousness: Its nature and functions* (chp. 12). Hauppauge, NY: Nova Publishers.

Segal, S.J. and Fusella, V. (1971). Effects of images in six sense modalities on detection of visual signal from noise. *Psychonomic Science*, 24, 55-56.

Schwamborn, A., Thillmann, H., Opfermann, M., and Leutner, D. (2011). Cognitive load and instructionally supported learning with provided and learner-generated visualizations. *Computers in Human Behavior*, 27, 89-93.

Schneider, J., Smith, W., and Whitcher, S. (1984, October). The relationship of mental imagery to white blood cell (neutrophil) function in normal subjects. *Paper presented at the 36th Annual Scientific Meeting of the International Society for Clinical and Experimental Hypnosis,* San Antonio, TX.

Shepard, R. N., and Metzler, J. (1971) Mental rotation of three-dimensional objects. *Science*, 171, 701-703.

Singer, D.G., Singer, J.L. (1990). The house of make-believe: Children's play and the developing imagination. Massachusetts: Harvard University Press.

Spiegel, D., and Moore, R. (1997). Imagery and hypnosis in the treatment of cancer patients. *Oncology*, 11, 1179-1189.

Stein, T.R., Olivo, E.L., Grand, S.H., Namerow, P.B., Costa, J., and Oz, M.C. (2010). A pilot study to assess the effects of a GI audiotape intervention on psychological outcomes in patients undergoing coronary artery bypass graft surgery. *Holistic Nursing Practice*, 24, 213-222.

Suk, M., Oh, W., and Kil, S. (2006). Guided imagery types on stress and performance of an intramuscular injection of nursing students. *Journal of Korean Academy of Nursing*, 36, 976-982.

Taylor, S. E., Pham, L. B., Rivkin, I. D., and Armor, D. A. (1998). Harnessing the imagination. *American Psychological Association*, 53, 429-439.

Tom, A. C., and Tversky, B. (2012). Remembering routes: Streets and landmarks. *Applied Cognitive Psychology*, 26, 182-193.

Trakhtenberg, E.C. (2008). The effects of guided imagery on the immune system: a critical review. *International Journal of Neuroscience*, 118 (6), 839-855.

Urech, C., Fink, N.S., Hoesli, I., Wilhelm, F.H., Bitzer, J., and Alder J. (2010). Effects of relaxation on psychobiological wellbeing during pregnancy: a randomized controlled trial. *Psychoneuroendocrinology*, 35, 1348-1355.

Walker, L.G., Walker, M.B., Ogston, K., Heys, S.D., Ah-See, A.K., Miller, I.D., Hutcheon, A.W., Sarkar, T.K., and Eremin, O. (1999). Psychological, clinical and pathological effects of relaxation training and guided imagery during primary chemotherapy. *British Journal of Cancer*, 80, 262-268.

Weigensberg, M.J., Lane, C.J., Winners, O., Wright, T., Nguyen-Rodriguez, S., Goran, M.I., and Spruijt-Metz, D. (2009). Acute effects of stress-reduction Interactive Guided Imagery(SM) on salivary cortisol in overweight Latino adolescents. *Journal Of Alternative and Complementary Medicine*, 15, 297-303.

West, T. G. (2009). In the mind's eye: Creative visual thinkers, gifted dyslexics and the rise of visual technologies (2nd ed.). New York: Prometheus Books.

Winnicott , D. (1971) Play and reality. London: Tavistock Publications.

Yoo, H.J., Ahn, S.H., Kim, S.B., Kim, W.K., and Han, O.S. (2005). Efficacy of progressive muscle relaxation training and GI in reducing chemotherapy side effects in patients with breast cancer and in improving their quality of life. *Supportive Care in Cancer*, 13, 826-833.

Zachariae, R., Kristensen, J.S., Hokland, P., Ellegaard, J., Metze, E., and Hokland, M. (1990). Effect of psychological intervention in the form of relaxation and GI on cellular immune function in normal healthy subjects. An overview. *Psychotherapy and Psychosomatics*, 54, 32-39.

Zachariae, R., Hansen, J.B., Andersen, M., Jinquan, T., Petersen, K.S., Simonsen, C., Zachariae, C., and Thestrup-Pedersen, K. (1994). Changes in cellular immune function after immune specific GI and relaxation in high and low hypnotizable healthy subjects. *Psychotherapy and Psychosomatics*, 61, 74-92.

Zachariae, R., Bjerring, P., and Arendt-Nielsen, L. (2007). Modulation of type I immediate and type VI delayed immunoreactivity using direct suggestion and GI during hypnosis. *Allergy*, 44, 537-542.

In: Alternative Medicine   ISBN 978-1-62257-106-2
Editors: Kenneth R. Carter and George E. Murphy   ©2012 Nova Science Publishers, Inc.

Chapter 2

REFLEXOLOGY - SCIENCE OR BELIEF

Jenny Jones[*,1] *and Stephen J. Leslie*[1,2]

[1]School of Nursing, Midwifery & Health, University of Stirling, Inverness, UK
[2]Highland Heartbeat Centre, Cardiology Unit, Raigmore Hospital, Inverness, UK

ABSTRACT

The use of complementary and alternative therapies, even in western industrialised countries with well developed conventional health care systems, ranges from 10-52%. Annual expenditure on complementary and alternative medicine (CAM) in the UK alone is estimated to be in excess of £1.6 billion. Despite this extensive use, complementary and alternative therapies have recently come under scrutiny in terms of their safety and efficacy, particularly in relation to claims made by practitioners. To date, robust scientific evidence for health benefit has been lacking for many alternative therapies, but despite this they remain popular.

Reflexology therapy is a form of sophisticated manual pressure applied most typically to the feet. It is one of the top six complementary and alternative therapies purchased. It is distinct from general massage due to two key therapeutic claims. First, that distinct areas on the feet correspond to specific internal organs within the body. Second, that massage to these discreet areas affects the haemodynamic status of the referred or 'mapped' organs in the body.

This chapter will describe and discuss in detail the basis for these haemodynamic theories by reviewing the original work of William H Fitzgerald and Eunice Ingham. The chapter will finish by describing the available contemporary evidence to support these theories and discusses the challenge of proving specific treatment effects in CAM in this current era of evidence-based medicine.

---

[*] Corresponding Author. Email: jenny.jones@stir.ac.uk; Tel: ++ 44 1463 255638; Fax: ++ 44 1463 255638.

INTRODUCTION

Reflexology is a complex massage intervention, based on the idea that specific areas on the soles of the feet (called reflex points), correspond or 'map' to individual internal organs in the body. Each organ is represented by a unique reflex point [1]. Reflexologists learn the location of these points from reflexology foot maps or charts. Eunice ngham invented the concept of reflexology in the 1930's and since then, it has gone on to become a hugely popular form of complementary therapy. Ingham made the claim that the application of reflexology massage to reflex points on the feet increases blood supply to the corresponding mapped organs in the body [2]. In her teachings, the reflexology haemodynamic treatment-related effect is believed to be quite distinct from non-specific foot massage components, such as simple touch, therapeutic exchange and placebo effects, even though these components can themselves cause haemodynamic responses [3-6].

Ingham's idea of a two-way relationship between specific points or areas of the feet and the organs of the body continues to dominate contemporary reflexology practice through the curriculum of the International Institute of Reflexology. This training organisation is the largest global provider of reflexology training and offers training based exclusively and explicitly on Ingham's theories [7]. The IIR deliver their training courses through 11 global franchised training branches [8] and claim to have at trained 25,000 reflexologists worldwide [9]. They remain the largest UK reflexology training provider [10].

Worldwide expenditure on CAM is estimated to be at least $40 billion per annum [11], with £1.6 billion spent annually in the UK alone [12;13]. Reflexology enjoys considerable public investment, particularly in Norway [14], Denmark [15] and the UK [12;16], where it is in the top six CAM therapies purchased. Individual reflexology sessions can cost from £15 (€18) - £70 (€84) per treatment and typically, 6-8 sessions are usually recommended by therapists to in order to gain the optimal therapeutic results [17;18]. Therefore the cost of an eight-week series could easily be in excess of £400 (€480) if an average of £50 (€60) per session is paid. Costs of up to £1000 (€1195) per year for repeated blocks of treatment may not be unusual for a patient with chronic health issues [19].

Due to this public-driven investment, reflexology safety and product quality have become healthcare research priorities [20], particularly in relation to the unique therapeutic claim of a specific haemodynamic effect. Any therapy that makes such a definable (and testable) prediction as this, evidence should be available to provide evidence to demonstrate that the product delivers as claimed and if it does, that the specific effect is safe and effective for all its users. This is particularly true for patient groups who may potentially be at risk from adverse treatment-related effects [21]. General adverse effects may include both intrinsic safety issues such as treatment errors or contraindications and extrinsic quality issues such as poor standardisation or quality control of the treatment delivered [20]. In the case of reflexology, if there is a significant specific haemodynamic effect, this raises particular questions about the intrinsic safety of the therapy for patients who may be adversely affected by an unanticipated change in haemodynamic status, such as those with heart disease [22]. Some cardiologists have voiced concerns that cardiovascular disease patients may be particularly vulnerable to the effects of CAM in general due to drug interaction, reduced adherence to conventional therapies or potential adverse effects amplified by the lack of CAM product standardisation [22]. An example of such an effect in relation to reflexology would be an arbitrary reflexology-induced change in haemodynamic status, which may be beneficial, but may also have an adverse effect.

To date, not one published reflexology research experiment has recruited from the cardiac patient population, so its effect on this patient group is unknown. Furthermore, only a few reflexology studies have controlled for non-specific effects in order to isolate any specific active component, despite the haemodynamic claim being a key part of the therapeutic value of reflexology. Thus, some doubt must remain over the validity of the haemodynamic claim. Furthermore, reflexology literature and teaching are inconsistent on the subject of the appropriateness of reflexology for cardiac patients. 'Heart or circulatory problems' are described as both an indication [23;24] and as a contraindication where treatment should be avoided [25-28]. It is reported that the haemodynamic effect of reflexology can adversely stress the cardiovascular system and potentially affect patients with mechanical implants such as pacemakers and artificial heart valves [29]. There is also a lack of consensus in the contemporary reflexology teaching literature about whether treatment to the heart reflex point itself carries with it the risk of a potential adverse-specific treatment effect, particularly for cardiac patients.

Despite its international popularity, Reflexology is a relatively recent therapeutic invention, which makes it unusual in CAM terms. Most CAM therapies are based on traditional beliefs, theories and cultural meaning of various indigenous populations, most typically Asian, African or Eastern, and have been used in these communities often for thousands of years [30]. Whereas the first documented appearance of the theory that provided the foundation for reflexology appeared relatively recently, its novel concepts detailed in two books, published in early twentieth century America. This recent history allows a unique opportunity to examine the therapeutic claims right from inception to present, in order to determine the quality of consistency of its historical narrative. Also, to more fully understand the exact nature of its inventors claims and to identify what component of the reflexology haemodynamic claim is experimentally falsifiable from within its own construct. This is possible because the entire foundational theory of contemporary reflexology is based purely on the therapeutic assumptions of two early twentieth century American healthcare professionals, Dr William Fitzgerald and physiotherapist Eunice Ingham.

This chapter will analyse these two historical texts and compare the theories and claims of the two authors with more recent reflexology literature. The comparative analysis between its foundational theories and contemporary interpretations will have a particular focus on the inconsistent reflexology opinions regarding the appropriateness of treatment for cardiac patients, in order to identify if there is any common framework that exists in the reflexology narrative. The chapter will conclude by discussing the significant methodological challenges facing researchers who aim to investigate the acute (immediate) haemodynamic effects of reflexology in cardiac patients and describe the methods we used in an attempt to overcome these challenges.

The Historical Origins of Reflexology and its Claim of a Specific Haemodynamic Effect

The entire foundational theory of contemporary reflexology is based on the therapeutic assumptions of two early twentieth century American healthcare professionals, Dr William Fitzgerald and physiotherapist Eunice Ingham.

Zone Therapy – For doctors only 185

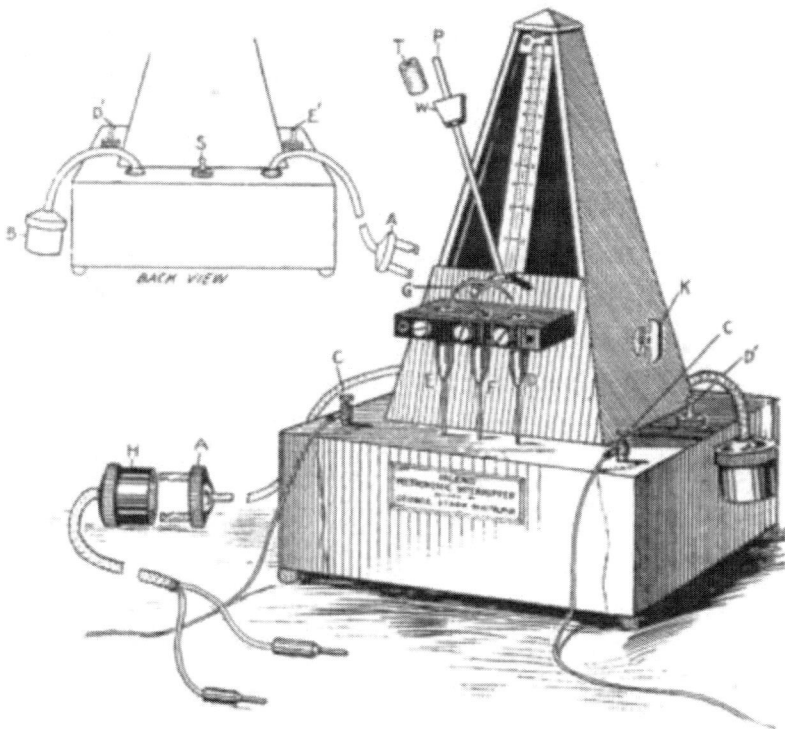

Valens Metronomic Interrupter (Style D)
(For Producing Dr. White's Pulsoidal Current)

Dr. William H. Fitzgerald

Dr William H Fitzgerald was the originator of the distinct theory that forms the basis for modern-day reflexology. He was an early twentieth century graduate of the Medical School of University of Vermont and worked as a surgeon in Boston City hospital, Central London Nose and Throat Hospital and as an otologist in Vienna [26]. Fitzgerald's medical training should have given him some awareness of the conditions necessary to scientifically justify claims of knowledge beyond observational induction, as concepts of deductive reasoning, statistics, inference, and blinded, controlled randomised experiments had already been well formulated by scientists such as Newton, Hume and Peirce [33].

FITZGERALD'S HYPOTHESIS

In 1912, during his tenure as head and surgeon of the Nose and Throat Department of St Francis Hospital in Hartford, Connecticut, Fitzgerald claimed to have accidentally discovered that pressure on the muco-cutaneus margin (where the skin joins the mucus membrane of the nose) – resulted in an anaesthetic effect as powerful as cocaine. As this simple action seemed to him to yield extraordinary results, he spent the next six years experimenting further, applying various forms of pressure to external peripheral areas all over the human body [31;32]. This experimentation led him to devise a theory about how certain aspects of the human body worked. Fitzgerald's ideas were based on his clinical observations of human reflex responses to pain or emotional distress. He interpreted unconscious reflex actions such as the gritting of teeth when in pain, clasping of an injured limb, gripping of a chair when frightened or in agony, the clenching the fists when in a state of anger and the clasping of hands when emotionally bereft, as signs that humans display a native involuntary urge to apply external pressure on the skin in times of pain, with the aim of producing an innate analgesic effect [33]. Based on these observations, Fitzgerald proposed that that the human automatic response to pain stimulus was specifically designed to stimulate a natural condition of anaesthesia within the body [34]. After further experimentation, he hypothesised that sustained and directed (non-accidental) pressure on distinct external areas of the human body also 'cured' various forms of underlying illness or disease in the internal body region below [35-41]. He defined this new theory as "a science" and named it Zone Therapy [33].

OUTLINE FOR STRUCTURAL ANALYSIS

The Conceptual Claims

Fitzgerald's theory proposes that the body is divided into ten longitudinal zone areas (Figure 1.1) and its effectiveness is based on certain assumptions. [32,33]

- There are five zones on either side of a central median line which run down the middle of the body
- Each zone related to the relevant fingers and toes of the body. The outer-most zone encompasses the thumb, extends up the arm through to the head and down to the greater toe. The second zone relates to the second finger and second toe using the same vertical longitudinal shape and so on
- Each zone is of equal width
- The tongue is also divided into ten zones, with the dorsal (top) surface corresponding to the anterior (front) sections of the body zones and the tongue as a whole, corresponding to the zones throughout the body
- The hard and soft palate and posterior walls of the pharynx and epipharynx are divided in the same way
- All body parts found in each zone are interlinked, which means that pain or disease in any one part potentially affects the rest of the zone

- The teeth reflect the innermost parts of every bone in the body and to a lesser extent, the tissues within all body zones, therefore all bones and related tissues in the body are reflected in the teeth
- Any inflammatory processes or injury on the periphery of the body such as the teeth, fingers or toes may excite, or be responsible for, disease or inflammation throughout any part of the internal related zone
- Any internal inflammatory disease processes within a given zone may be responsible for peripheral inflammatory imbalances or symptoms in the teeth, fingers, toes or tongue

Based on these assumptions, his theory predicts the following causal links between the considered application of pressure, and changes in the human condition, that are not normally biologically and causally linked with direct (non-accidental) pressure [33;34;42;43]:

a. The conscious application of a sustained, direct (non-accidental) pressure to external accessible area of each zone will specifically affect all inaccessible inner body parts in the same zone
b. Following the application of sustained (non-accidental) pressure on an external part of a zone, a form of natural endogenous analgesia will occur within the corresponding internal regions of the corresponding zone
c. If the pressure is applied firmly enough and for long enough, it produces a condition of anaesthesia more potent than opiates, therefore can be used in place of anaesthetic to induce a pain-free state in which minor surgical operations can be successfully carried out
d. Applied pressure will also cause lymphatic relaxation and result in the lymph being stimulated to flow normally in its channels
e. The correct application of zone therapy will not only relieve pain, but will often remove the cause of the pain, regardless of underlying pathology
f. Therefore the application of direct (non-accidental) pressure is never arbitrary or harmful, it is always therapeutically beneficial

Mode of Activation

Fitzgerald developed a variety of tools to apply the correct 'dosage' of external pressure on various periphery of the body. Pressure was reportedly applied from one-half minute to up to four minutes on average and recommended to be as deep and firm as the receiver could bear it [33].The instruments he used ranged from clothes pegs or elastic bands wrapped tight around the finger tips (Figure 2), metal combs grasped tightly in a clenched hand, nasal probes pressed inside the naval cavity or probes firmly pressed upon the surface of the tongue or soft palate (Figure 3). Distinct peripheral areas were selected for treatment in relation to their proximity to the condition or disease in the underlying corresponding zone. Other times, areas were identified if they were deemed to be presenting localised symptoms that had manifested from internal disease in the corresponding zone. In particular, as the tongue and teeth were regarded as being able to affect or reflect the innermost parts of all zones, prolonged teeth clamping or tongue compression was often advised, in fact Fitzgerald devotes an entire chapter of his book for use by dentists [44].

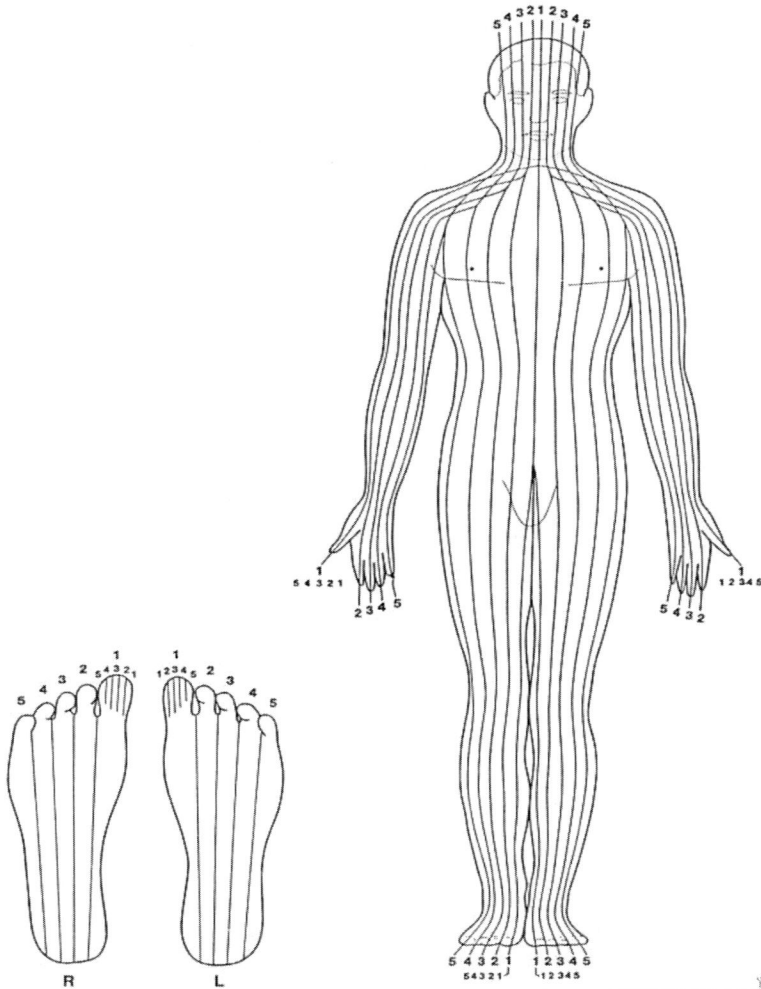

Figure 1. Fitzgerald's conceptual model - the body is divided into ten longitudinal zone areas.

Theories of Causality

In 1917, Fitzgerald and Dr Edwin F Bowers, another zone therapy advocate, published a book of first-hand accounts of case studies entitled "Zone Therapy or Relieving Pain at Home" [45]. Throughout his writing, Fitzgerald speculated about several mechanisms of action to explain his ideas, which can be broadly categorised as either materialist (having physical/biological form) or immaterialist, (appealing to non-material phenomena e.g. healing power of nature).

Making the deaf hear 59

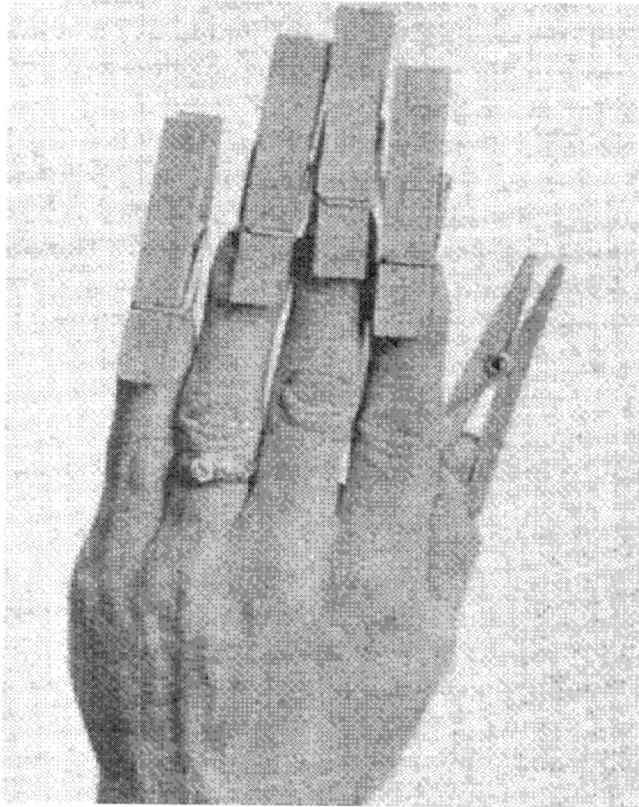

Figure 2. Adapted, hollowed-out clothes pegs used to apply pressure to the fingers for the relief of pain, to desensitise the teeth for dental operations, and to make the deaf hear.

Materialist Mechanisms

He considered "blocked shock" or "nerve block" as one potential mechanism and hypothesised that applied pressure to the nerves running from an injured extremity to the brain potentially *"inhibits or prevents the transmission to the brain, the knowledge of injury"* by inducing a state of inhibition in the relevant zone nerve impulses [33]. However the seemingly unrelated locations of applied pressure in some of his case studies seemed to contradict this premise. He also linked zone therapy pressure with lymphatic relaxation and flow stimulation and proposed that many pathological conditions disappeared as a result [33], but it is unclear whether he regarded the simulation of lymph flow as the key causal agent in treatment-related disease remission. He also speculated briefly about Bowers hypothesis, which suggested the existence of ultra-microscopic connections, analogous to the pathways of the nervous system [34], but this explanation had fundamental flaws, as Fitzgerald offered no biologically plausible explanation as to the means these ultra-microscopic connections might use to interface with the underlying physiology in order to bring about a referred analgesic condition or disease remission state (Figure 4).

48   ZONE THERAPY.

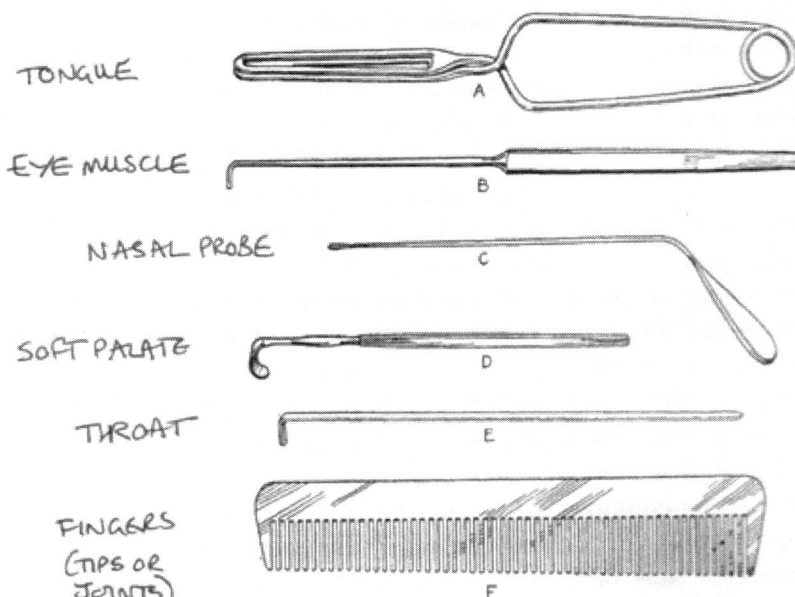

TONGUE — A

EYE MUSCLE — B

NASAL PROBE — C

SOFT PALATE — D

THROAT — E

FINGERS (TIPS OR JOINTS) — F

Non-Electrical Applicators Useful in Zone Therapy

A is an ordinary surgical clamp which can be used for clamping the tongue.

B is an ordinary eye-muscle retractor. This can be used for intermittently retracting the posterior pillars of the fauces.

C is a special type of nasal probe used for attacking the posterior wall of the nasopharynx.

D is a regular palpebral retractor which can be used for intermittently retracting the soft palate, especially in the region of the fossa of Rosenmüller.

E is a regular flat applicator bent up at one end. This is useful about the throat and fauces. It can be used as a pressure applicator for the posterior wall of the oropharynx.

F is an ordinary aluminum comb used for attacking the fingers or toes either at the tips or about the joints.

Figure 3. Non-electrical applicators used by Fitzgerald to apply pressure on various peripheral surfaces of the body.

Several problems arise from Fitzgerald's materialist theories. First, he gives no logical explanation as to how such profound physiological change can be causally bought into being, purely by the act of directed (non-accidental) pressure to the periphery of the body, other than the volitional intention of the zone therapist for it to do so. Second, he offered no explanation as to how external physical pressure could interface with, or translate to, the internal physiological systems of the human body in order to control the complex involuntary, numerous physiological processes necessary to regulate disease remission or profound states of analgesia to order. And third, he fails to explain how the specific effect arising from applied, distinct external pressure could distinguish random or 'accidental' pressure that is exerted on the body by clothes, close proximity to another, supportive furniture such as chairs, shoes, the ground underneath the feet etc., compared to sustained and directed (non-accidental) applied pressure of zone therapy. Similar problems are also evident in his immaterialist theories of causality.

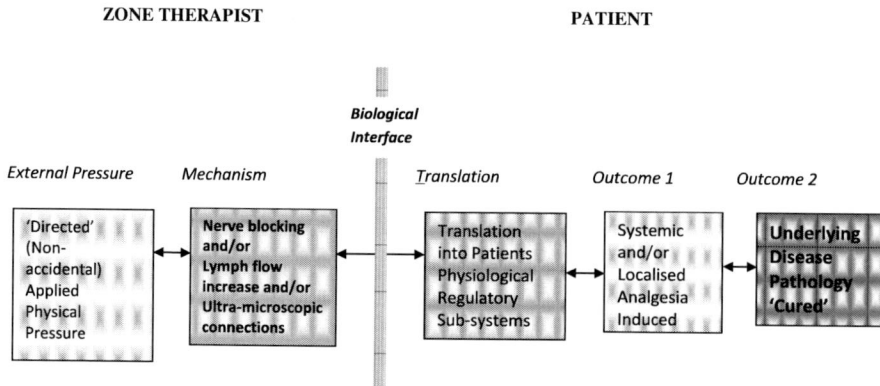

Figure 4. Schematic illustrating Fitzgerald's hypothesised materialist mechanisms of action, operating via a biological interface - interacting with the patient's physiological matter.

Immaterial Mechanisms

In order to produce complex effects such as disease remission or healing, zone therapy also needed to appeal to immaterial forces such as the healing power of nature, the "*Cosmic Force that envelopes us all in a mantle of kindness and love*" [46] or at other times, the "*soothing influence of animal magnetism*" [34]. This referred to a supposed magnetic fluid or ethereal medium which was believed to exist inside the bodies of animate (breathing) beings, which could be wilfully manipulated by the careful laying on of hands [47] or in the case of zone therapy, direct (non-accidental) applied pressure [33]. 'Nature' or Cosmic Forces, were also seen as an active agents, operating as beneficent organising agencies, capable of restoring the body to full health when stimulated by some form of operator (in this case the therapist applying specific directed pressure). Fitzgerald's presumption that these unquantifiable forces could be stimulated to act, implied that in his model, 'Nature' / Cosmic Forces are somehow malleable but dormant, waiting passively for someone to operationalize either in order to restore normal pathology in the presence of disease.This apparent ambivalent passivity of Nature / Cosmic Forces in the face of underlying disease pathology would seem to be somewhat at odds with Fitzgerald's notions of these immaterial entities being inherently benevolent, once activated (Figure 5).

Other fundamental problems that applied to his materialist interpretation also apply equally to his notions of immaterialist phenomena. For instance, Fitzgerald gives no explanation as to how these immaterial phenomena interface with, or translate to, material or physical matter in order to control the complex involuntary, numerous physiological processes necessary in order to regulate disease remission to order. Second, he gives no logical explanation as to how these immaterial phenomena can be made manifest purely by the act of directed applied pressure to the periphery of the body. Furthermore, how the immaterial agency distinguishes random or 'accidental' pressure that is exerted on the body by clothes, close proximity to another, supportive furniture such as chairs, shoes, the ground underneath the feet etc., compared to directed (non-accidental) applied pressure.

IMMATERIAL TO MATERIAL

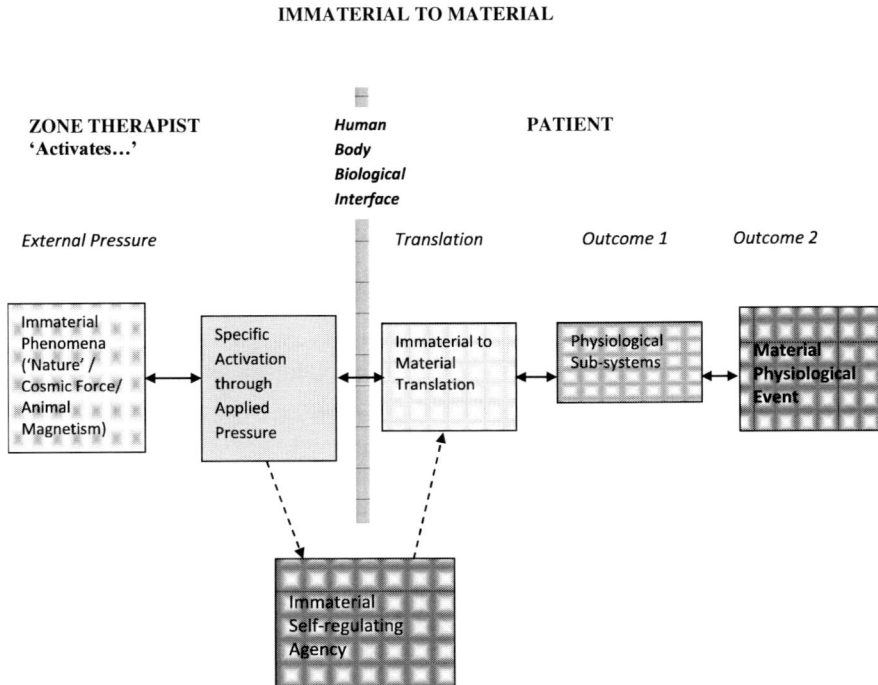

Figure 5. Schematic illustrating Fitzgerald's hypothesised immaterial phenomena of action, operating via unknown interface - interacting with patient's physiological matter.

In effect, it appears from his writing that Fitzgerald expected an effect out of zone therapy, and believed he got what he expected. However he appeared to have made no methodological efforts to control for non-specific effects such as suggestibility, placebo, simple regression to the mean, misdiagnosis or spontaneous recovery in his subjects [48], even though the concept of suggestibility in a medical context was already being widely discussed in early twentieth century medical and popular literature

Zone Therapy's Relevance to Specific Haemodynamic Effect Claim and Treatment Strategies for Patients with Heart Disease

Fitzgerald makes only passing reference to one form of acute cardiovascular event, chest pain, and suggests that if it remains unrelieved by applied zone pressure, the pain is due to abnormal pressure being applied from within the zone itself, such as

"irritation, gas, pus, impactions, or necrosis, all of which demand immediate medical attention" [33].

However there is no mention in Fitzgerald's writing of a specific haemodynamic effect being causally linked to applied zone therapy pressure treatment. His only reference to any kind of haemodynamic component is non-specific, when he advises against the constriction of blood vessels by "undue irritation of the nerve zones" [33] caused by excessive pressure of tight belts, corsets or collars. But he does not distinguish how the effects of abnormal pressure such as clothing restriction can be distinguished from the proposed beneficial effects of applied zone therapy pressure. Apart from these two brief asides, he offers no case study examples of the treatment of any degree of heart disease in his writing. After publication of his first book, he did not appear to publish further on zone therapy, and there is little evidence of his subsequent activities in the field.

Eunice Ingham

Eunice Ingham was a physiotherapist in the early 1930's. After learning zone therapy from a student of Fitzgerald's, Ingham made several crucial amendments to its theory and practice and distinguished her version of the therapy by naming it reflexology. She offered no logical justification for these changes, therefore the remodelling of Fitzgerald's zone therapy appeared to be based on personal belief.

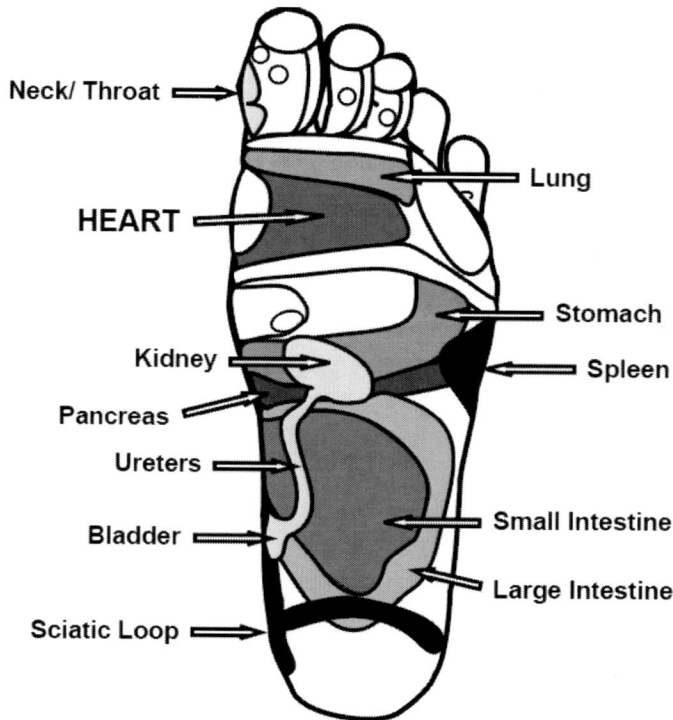

Figure 6. Inghams Reflexology Chart of the feet showing the various organ reflex areas. (Original artwork; **David Ditchfield**)

Ingham's Hypothesis

Ingham made a finite set of observations arising from her own self-reported experimentation with zone therapy and from these results and her own personal beliefs, devised her theory of how the body worked. Ingham decided that the soles of the feet represent a proportional scaled map of the major organs and internal body parts and this correspondence is biologically fundamental to the design of the human body. Furthermore, she believed there were discreet, two-way feedback loops between each individual organ and corresponding areas on the feet (Figure 6), areas which she labelled as reflex points   [49]. For her, reflexology relied on the following assumptions, some shared with Fitzgerald's concept, some entirely distinct to her own model:

OUTLINE FOR STRUCTURAL ANALYSIS

The Conceptual Claims

1. There are five zones on either side of a central median line which run down the middle of the body [50]
2. Each zone related to the relevant fingers and toes of the body. The outer-most zone encompasses the thumb, extends up the arm through to the head and down to the greater toe. The second zone relates to the second finger and second toe using the same vertical longitudinal shape and so on [51].
3. Each zone is of equal width [51]
4. The feet are the most sensitive external zone area of the body [31]
5. The feet offer a perfect scaled-down representational model template of the human body, with the toes representing the head, the ball of the foot the upper part of the body, and the heel representing body parts below the waist (Figure 1.9) [51]
6. The precise location of the organ or body part mapping on the soles of the feet represents a collection of unique and individual discreet areas of nerve endings or reflexes in each discreet area [52]
7. The body is constantly in motion, with the "*natural muscular activity of each organ keeping its whole nerve canal free from detrimental obstruction*" [52]
8. Each reflex area therefore corresponds exclusively with its corresponding mapped organ or distal body part in the body via means of a discreet feedback loop [52;53]
9. Aspects of this interconnectedness rely on the "*22 miles of tubing*" that makes up the blood stream and corresponding "*nerve endings*" and capillaries in the feet [54]
10. This blood and reflex interconnectedness allows a diagnostic corresponding representation of disease in the distal organ or body part to manifest in the distinct reflex area of either foot [50;51;55].

Ingham's theory allowed her to propose novel explanations about the cause and nature of ill health, one form originating from the periphery, the other from an internal source; in effect, she proposed a top-down or bottom-up approach to the formation of disease, which can be summarised in the following model-dependant assumptions. First, she theorised that disease could be caused by degenerative muscle weakening of the feet. In this respect, her first theory sees the causal nature of disease being directly related to the condition of the feet, put simply, she saw disease as being caused by a 'foot up' influence [50]:

In this model, as body muscle generally weakens, the feet muscles weaken also. This results in misplaced foot joints. Misplaced joints then place undue pressure on certain nerve endings. Each discreet nerve ending is part of a unique individual feedback loop with a corresponding or 'mapped' individual organ or distal body part. The undue pressure shuts off normal 'nerve' and blood supply in the feet, resulting in the circulating blood stream corresponding to the discreet feedback loop between the nerve ending and associated body part becoming blocked or stagnated. This slows down circulation in the discreet feedback loop and allows formation of chemical deposits/toxic waste matter around misplaced foot joints or nerves. The corresponding organ nerves are then affected by the peripheral nerve clogging process. This interruption in the clear circulation of individual feedback loops interferes with the "proper contraction and relaxation" of the corresponding organ, which results in the organ failing to get a sufficient 'fresh supply of blood'. The feedback loop circulation stagnation or sluggishness means that the referred organ then loses its ability to eliminate waste matter, e.g. Kidneys unable to eliminate uric acid sufficiently. Gravity then forces the waste matter deposits or 'toxins' to settle in the feet within the discreet feedback loop around the corresponding nerve reflex area.

Her other notion of disease causality involved ideas of inherited or constitutional organ or body weakness, which in her model, manifests in the feet by causing corresponding imbalances or weakness in the relevant reflex point area [50]. In this theory, any inherited or constitutional weakness in organ or body part results in the organs being unable to perform *"proper contraction and relaxation"* activity [52]. This results in insufficient force of circulation to keep the reflected nerve ending in the associated discreet feedback loop, free of waste matter. Then, as waste matter accumulates in the referred foot area of the circulatory feedback loop, the related organ suffers greater blood circulation loss and increase in toxic waste matter build up.

Based on these assumptions of the origin of disease and foot disorders, Ingham's theory predicts the following specific relationship between the application of reflexology pressure techniques, and changes in the human condition, that are not normally biologically and causally linked with direct (non-accidental) pressure:

a.   Signs of toxin aggregation in the form of 'grittiness' (a sense of 'crystals' under the planter skin of the sole of the foot) or tender foot areas evidence a 'sluggish' circulation within an individual feedback loop [55]

b.   These crystals suggest either a localised peripheral imbalance, or a state of imbalance in the corresponding reflected body area or organ [55]

c.   By palpating the soles of the feet and massaging these gritty or tender foot areas using touch techniques unique to Ingham's model, the congestive toxic deposits in the circulating feedback loop will be broken down in the nerve reflex areas, clearing the obstruction [55]

d.   As nerve-endings or reflexes in the feet organs are mapped to referred body parts via 'nerve canals' or discreet individual circulatory feedback loops, the circulation to the corresponding organ will improve as a result [55]

e.   The massage dissolves the waste matter so that normal circulation can be restored both to the nerve reflex areas and to the referred organ [55]

f.   "Nature" can then repair whatever may have caused the imbalance in the first place [24]

g.   *"The more of this toxic material the blood contains, the more severe will be the reaction...this is nature's way of cleaning house and eliminating the poisons from the system"* [55]

Mode of Activation

Ingham changed the physical touch pressure technique from Fitzgerald's constant applied pressure to a form of distinct massage-touch techniques unique to reflexology, which she applied most typically to the feet. She described her technique as a "*slow creeping and slight pulling back movement*" [56]. She offered no logical justification for this treatment change in her books therefore the remodelling of Fitzgerald's techniques appeared to be based on nothing more than personal belief.

Theory of Causality

Ingham published two books, "Stories the Feet can Tell", in 1938, and "Stories the Feet Have Told" in 1951. These books have a seminal position in contemporary reflexology practice and form the core curriculum of the IIR training method [57]. Throughout her writing, Ingham proposed several mechanisms of action, which can be broadly categorised as either materialist (having physical/biological form), or immaterialist, (appealing to non-material phenomena). The mechanisms assumed in both will now be briefly discussed.

"Stories the Feet Can Tell" (1938)

In this book, it is clear from the very outset that Ingham's reflexology theory bore little resemblance to Fitzgerald's original zone therapy model. Although she still referred to the zone model as a viable therapeutic theory for the human body, she hypothesised that it is the feet that most reliably 'tell the story' of what is actually going on in the body [50]. This diagnostic capability depended on Ingham's idea that crystalline deposits or areas of tenderness found on the feet were the means by which ill-health or disease in individual organs generally materialised. She believed that if no tenderness or deposits were found in the heart reflex of a person medically diagnosed with heart disease, then the medical diagnosis was wrong [58]. And although the notion of the reflex points on the feet was a new core component of reflexology, Ingham appeared to arbitrarily change her meaning and usage of the word throughout her writing.

Material Causes

For material causation, Ingham introduced the idea of accumulating toxic 'crystalline' waste matter, which she believed 'settled' in the 'nerve endings' or reflex point found in the feet [50]. She asserted that as crystals blocked individual areas of peripheral nerve endings, then the associated nerves in the corresponding organ would become clogged, leading to the 'normal muscular activity' of the corresponding organ circulation becoming impaired, resulting in deceleration of the circulation of the blood through the affected organ [55].

This proposition was the first appearance of any suggestion of a two-way haemodynamic link in reflexology and appeared to rely on the idea that reflex areas of the feet have distinct feedback loops to individual organs via nerve channels (Figure 7).

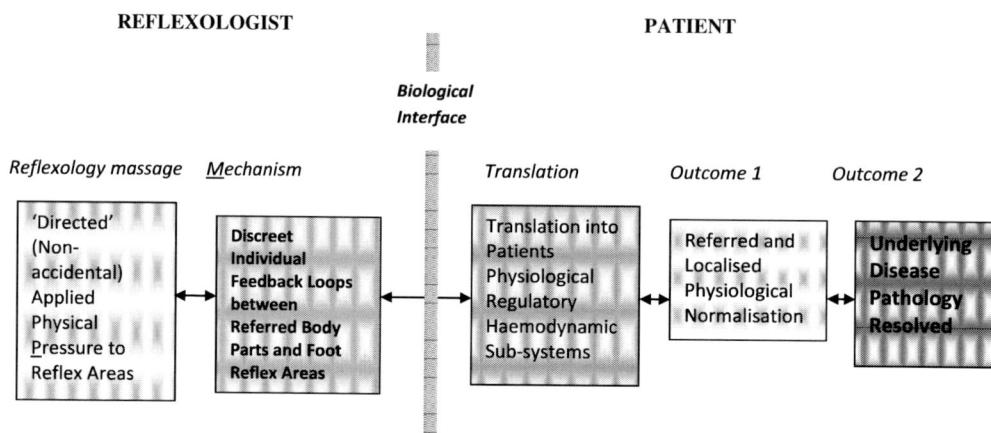

Figure 7. Schematic illustrating Ingham's hypothesised materialist mechanisms of action, operating via a biological interface - interacting with the patient's physiological matter.

Ingham also varied in her explanations of the nature of the crystals of toxic substances that she believed impeded the periphery of these feedback loops, describing them at various times as chemical deposits, poisonous acid, crystalline deposits or toxins [50]. She offered no explanation as to the origins of these toxins or specified the name of a single, identifiable chemical toxin which could be measured or extracted for testing, except for the occasional mention of 'calcium' deposits giving rise to 'acid' crystals [52]. Ingham's idea of 'toxins' is also problematic because any metabolic waste products from the tissues are washed out into the cardiovascular system for eventual filtration and excretion by the kidneys [59], but these metabolic waster products are not generally categorised as 'toxins' and there is no evidence that these materials crystallise and 'settle' in the nerve endings of the feet. So Ingham's idea of toxins arguably has no scientific meaning, even though she stated that the efficacy of reflexology was built on the opinions of practising physicians [60]. Second, if the 'toxins' such as 'acid crystals' settle in the feet due to gravity, then many other metabolic components must also 'settle' in the feet alongside the toxins, which means our feet would contain an inordinate amount of matter or material compared to the rest of the body.

IMMATERIAL CAUSES

Like Fitzgerald, she also appealed to an intangible agent she describes as 'nature' in her first book [55], which she seemed to regard as some kind of active agent, capable restoring the body to full health, but more so when wilfully stimulated by some form of operator (in this case the therapist) (Figure 8).

IMMATERIAL TO MATERIAL

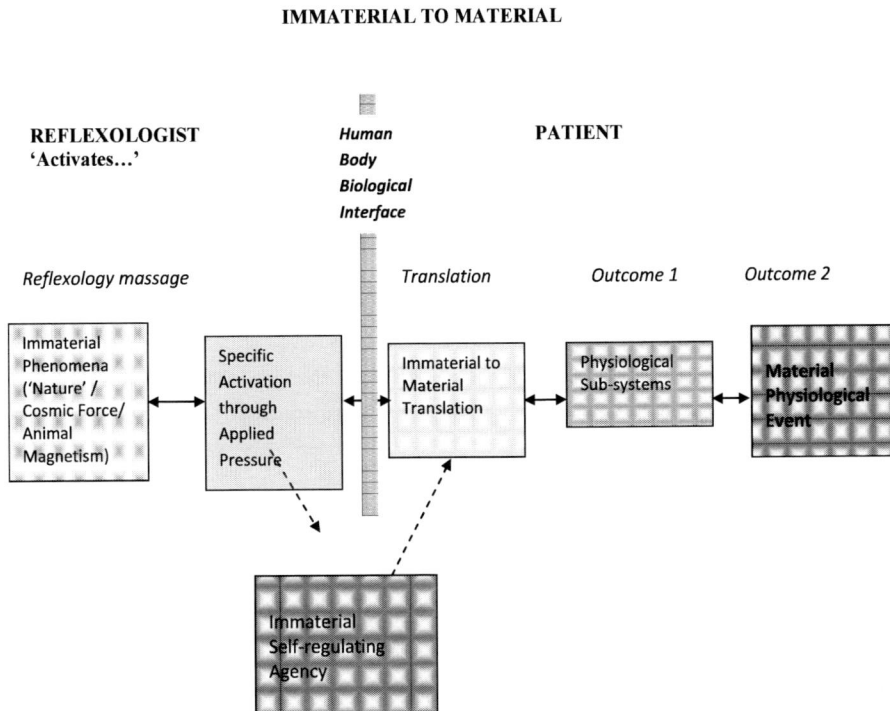

Figure 8. Schematic illustrating Ingham's hypothesised immaterial phenomena of action, operating via unknown interface - interacting with patient's physiological matter.

"Stories the Feet Have Told" (1951)

In her second book, Ingham seems to have re-interpreted her original notions of healing agency as an intangible etheric form in the body, and now described this healing energy as 'electro-mechanism', with the reflex points in the feet said to be acting as terminals for the flow [61]. In a chapter entitled "Terminals", she made an analogy between her hypothesised reflexes and the 'terminal' ends of the arteries, where they transform into veins, speculating that 'blockages' impeded the beneficial conduction of the electrical forces of the earth into the feet terminals [62]. Ingham still continued to evoke notions of 'nature' as a self-regulating agency but it is unclear whether she now believed 'electro-mechanism' was nature itself, or nature made manifest as a definable entity, or "*God's great infallible laws of nature*" [63;64]. Whatever her interpretation of its essence, she continued to move back and forth between concepts [61;65].

Although she presents her findings as fact throughout her two books and uses the word 'science' to describe reflexology on several occasions [66-68], Ingham had little awareness of the conditions necessary to scientifically justify claims of knowledge. She offered no experimental evidence except for her series of self-reported case studies. On this basis, her view that the theory of reflexology could be guaranteed by nothing more than a series of unfalsifiable conjectures and a finite number of observations which partially depended on appeals to immaterial properties for causality, raises questions about how she distinguished science from metaphysical forms of belief such as faith healing. Furthermore, like Fitzgerald, she appeared to have made no efforts to control for errors such as suggestibility, placebo, simple regression to the mean, misdiagnosis or spontaneous recovery as potential confounding factors in her interpretation of her treatment results [48], even though she herself acknowledges the role of suggestibility in disease causality [67].

Therapeutic Technique in Relation to Treating Patients with Various Degrees of Heart Disease

In her first book, Ingham described the anatomy of the heart, and then discussed the effects of 'congestion', which can be interpreted to be related to coronary artery disease. She suggested that any tenderness in the heart reflex zone area (located in the upper half of the left foot in her construct),was evidence of congestion in the arteries and veins surrounding the heart, which she proposed would eventually lead to life-threatening clots. She asserted that the heart must be

"... flushed with the proper blood supply, which you will be able to give it by freeing these nerve endings of all acid or calcium deposits where there is a tender reflex" [69].

She recommended that practitioners work the heart reflex area gently at first (if tender), but advises that they return to work on it two or three times during the treatment session, implying that more treatment is better than less. In cases of Angina Pectoris, she claims to have treated a number of cases very successfully and advised the following treatment strategy –

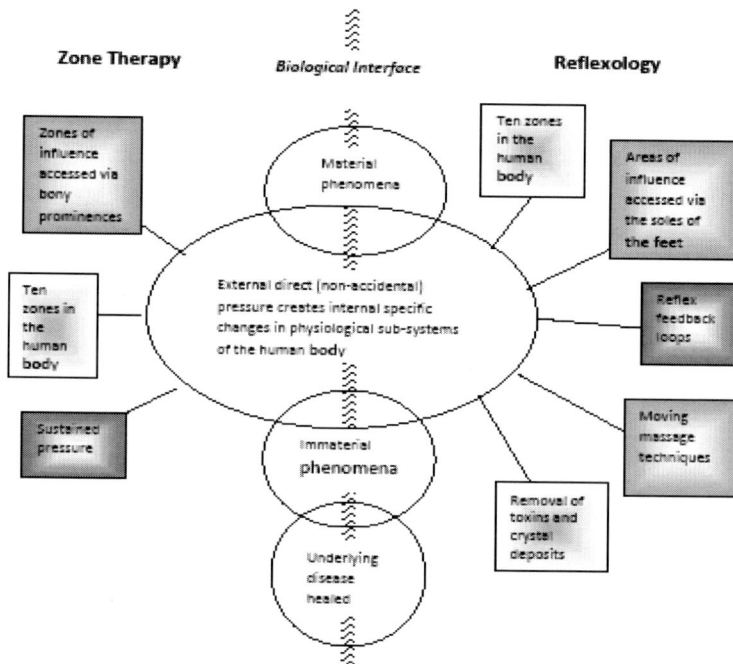

Figure 9. Schematic illustrating Fitzgerald's and Inghams shared and separate concepts.

"... if the pain extends up toward the shoulder and neck, work up towards the root of the fourth and fifth toes. Keep trying until you find the tenderness, then set to and work it out...you must work on the foot according to the location the pain around the heart. If the pain extends down toward the arm, work around the base of the little toe, as pointed out and directed for trouble in the shoulder. Since it is certain no harm can be done by working on a reflex, there is no need to hesitate, but set out and do all the good that can be accomplished" [69]

This clearly implies that she sees no harm in working the heart reflex area even in the presence of any gradation of heart disease. Furthermore, it appears that repeated work to the area during a treatment session is advised. In her second book, she refers to calcification of the arterial vessels as the key cause of high blood pressure, and cites the primary cause as faulty 'elimination' or tension often found following a 'distorted mental attitude' or 'mental stress' (although it is not clear whether she relates the calcium involved in hypertension to be the same calcium involved in her crystalline toxic deposit law). However in this book, she offers no direct treatment strategy for either, save for adopting a more cheerful countenance.

SUMMARY OF DIFFERENCES AND SIMILARITIES BETWEEN THE TWO THEORIES

Although there are some overlapping concepts between the two models, the operational and theoretical principles of each differ in substantial ways (Figure 9).

Both authors came to believe that a specific causal link existed between the application of direct (non-accidental) pressure techniques, and changes in the human condition, that are not normally biologically and causally linked with direct (non-accidental) pressure and second, the appeal by both to immaterial forces (including God) for causality. However, even in these two shared principles, there appears to be substantial differences in interpretation. Fitzgerald believed that the specific effect was evoked through sustained, prolonged pressure on the peripheral finger digits, the tongue and at other times, the soft palate. Whereas Ingham operationalised her effect through unique moving massage therapy techniques delivered to the soles and ankles of the feet. If she involved the hands at all, she used the palms, not the digits. She also proposed that the human body was somehow biologically mapped to the soles of the feet and invoked notions of toxins and discreet individual feedback loops of circulating blood between distinct areas of this map and individual corresponding organs as necessary components in this construct. Whereas Fitzgerald saw a broader body-wide zone-region construct, with no mention of discreet feedback loops or toxins. In fact, it seems that the only truly shared concept between the two models is the rather vague idea that necessitating causal links exist between the considered application of any form of pressure (be it moving massage or sustained), and specific beneficial changes in the human condition, which are not normally biologically and causally linked with any form of direct (non-accidental) pressure. However as the analysis indicated, neither author made any attempt to explain how 'directed' pressure as such could be differentiated between the normal physical pressure experienced in daily activities such as chewing, eating food which the tongue physically manipulates, standing (pressure on the back/sacral area), sitting (same), leaning against objects (pressure on relevant body area), walking (pressure on most areas of the soles of the feet), wearing clothes (shoes, belts, collars, etc), picking up objects (pressure on finger pads, palms etc), feeling things (same), etc. Ingham very briefly mentioned ill-fitting or constricting shoes leading to impediment of circulation in that corresponding reflex area   [51], but again, did not distinguish how her directed (non-accidental) pressure evoked a powerful positive healing response in the distal regions of the body whereas the accidental pressure applied by an ill-fitting shoe did not.

TREATMENT STRATEGIES AND THEORIES FOR CARDIAC PATIENTS

Both authors differ regarding treatment strategies for patients with various gradations of heart disease. As the analysis showed, Fitzgerald made no specific recommendations for treating cardiac disease; therefore the reflexology literature inconsistencies quoted in the chapter introduction would appear to have their origins in Ingham's work. Her law for treating patients with any gradation of heart disease can be categorised as a '*no therapy specific risk*' belief. In other words, she saw no harm in working on a reflex, regardless of the disease state of the corresponding organ. And even though her explanation of causality involved ideas of breaking up 'blockages' in the circulatory feedback loop system, she seemed to distinguish the desired intentional goal of dissolution of circulatory 'blockages' from the potentially hazardous biological interpretation which suggests dislodgement or break-up of a blood clot, which could then turn into a potentially life-threatening circulating embolus. In the case of treating the heart reflex area on cardiac patients, this would seem to suggest a product safety concern in Inghams highly popular commercial model, as over 2% of post-myocardial infarction (MI) patients present with clinically evident systematic embolisms and over 60% of patients with a large anterior MI have an increased risk of embolic thrombus [70], however she makes no reference to this increased risk amongst the cardiac patient population. This implies that she did not regard the 'blockages' as being material in nature, which seems somewhat inconsistent with other laws in her belief model, as she also proposed that the blockages (in the form of crystalline toxic deposits) were palpable on the soles of the feet.

IDENTIFICATION OF WHAT IS EXPERIMENTALLY FALSIFIABLE IN RELATION TO THE REFLEXOLOGY HAEMODYNAMIC EFFECT

Ingham consistently described the specific haemodynamic phenomenon in vague ways, lacking any clarity or detail as to the physical nature or biological scope of the effect, apart from fuzzy ideas that 'nerve' blockages impede blood circulation in the distinct feedback loop and removal of these blockages enables the corresponding organ to get "*a fresh supply of blood*" [52]. However the falsifiable condition in her theory is the idea that each organ of the body is part of a specific feedback loop which when activated, enables the relevant organ to receive 'more blood'. Regardless of the fact that the underlying causal mechanisms Ingham appeals to rely on unfalsifiable material and immaterial explanations of causality which include appeals to God, the outcome of a specific haemodynamic effect is a proposition that is experimentally testable.

EVIDENCE FOR THE HAEMODYNAMIC CLAIMS

Based on the idea that the specific haemodynamic effect is a proposition that can be tested, we performed a systematic evaluation of existing reflexology RCT's to determine whether there was any evidence to suggest the existence of a specific reflexology haemodynamic effect and if so, how it had been experimentally demonstrated? We identified only 48 randomised controlled trials of reflexology in the world literature available as full text [71]. Of these only 12 trials reported the effect on cardiac or vascular parameters [72-81]. However ten of the 12 studies delivered reflexology as a whole treatment, often using foot massage as a control treatment. Therefore it was not possible to determine the existence of any specific haemodynamic component in the therapy due to the fact that foot massage may have 'contaminated' the control by accidentally 'hitting' or massaging reflex points during the foot massage. Only two trials attempted to investigate the impact of touch as compared to the whole reflexology treatment. i.e. only two attempted to control for other non-specific effects of the therapy and in both cases, although the experimental methods were not entirely robust, their findings suggested the presence of a specific haemodynamic effect that was distinct from the non-specific effects generally associated with foot massage [80;81].

The results of the literature search confirmed that there was a clear need for research using a more innovative design and robust methods which could allow a specific haemodynamic effect to reveal itself, in order to provide high quality evidence to enable cardiac patients users to make a more informed decision about the safety and product quality of the haemodynamic claim. Overall, the literature findings highlighted three key methodological challenges that reflexology research designs need to overcome in order to be considered robust and reliable:

1. How to overcome the issue of inconsistent reflexology foot maps?
2. How to develop a simple standardised reflexology intervention?
3. How to devise a suitable form of control?

REFLEXOLOGY RESEARCH CHALLENGES

As we found a lack of rigorous evidence, we attempted to meet the research challenge of isolating a specific haemodynamic effect ourselves. First, in order to overcome the challenge of the variation in reflexology foot maps, we selected one reflex point for testing purposes to see if reflexology massage to this particular point would specifically affect the haemodynamic status of the corresponding mapped organ. Given the reflexology product safety concerns amongst the cardiac population, it seemed appropriate to pick the heart reflex point itself in order to determine whether causal links exist between the application of reflexology massage techniques to the heart reflex point and specific beneficial changes in the haemodynamic status of the heart. However, before attempting to design a reflexology intervention, we looked for guidance from the contemporary reflexology teaching literature in order to answer the following questions:

1. Do contemporary reflexology theorists and educators consider reflexology to be appropriate and safe for cardiac patients?
2. If so, what are the recommended heart reflex point treatment strategies for patients with cardiac disease?

To answer these questions, the dominant professional reflexology organisations and key commercial training providers were identified, so that only authorised and recommended versions of teaching material would be referenced.

ACCREDITED REFLEXOLOGY TEACHING LITERATURE

In line with many CAM therapies, reflexology is moving towards a more standardised training and educational structure. Professional reflexology training programs changed as a result of the House of Lords Select Committee report on CAM (2000), the Kings Fund Report (2008), Professor Stone's voluntary regulation proposals and the Federal Working Group recommendations [16;82-84]. The outcome of these enquiries led to the Complementary and Natural Healthcare Council (CNHC) being set up to regulate professional standards for a UK-wide voluntary register of CAM practitioners [85]. The CNHC aim is to protect the public by ensuring that CAM registrants meet minimum practitioner quality and product safety standards in their practice and the Department of Health recommend that the public use CNHC registered practitioners wherever possible [86]. Suitably qualified reflexologists are currently eligible for entry to the CNHC Register if they have completed a validated programme of education and gained professional registration status which meets the CNHC requirements [87]. If the practitioner applies for CNHC registration, they are obliged to continue a set amount of professional development training every year. Membership of the CNHC means that the reflexology profession is more open to public scrutiny, but at the same time, it is a form of guarantee to the public that the reflexologist has achieved an approved level of training and this training has been recognised as being of professional standard. Registration of the CNHC is voluntary at this time, but it is generally assumed that membership will become mandatory in due course.

The CNHC currently recognises three professional reflexology associations in the UK which exist to represent the interests of professional reflexologists. These are the British Reflexology Association (BRA), the International Federation of Reflexologists (IFR) and the Association of Reflexologists (AoR). These member associations sit within the larger Reflexology Forum council, a top-level organisation which operates as a voluntary overall regulator of the profession. In 2004, in line with the CNHC requirements for standardisation of training, the Reflexology Forum developed a set of common standards for the practice and training of reflexology. These standards now form the "core curriculum" of reflexology training and are based on the National Occupational Standards set down by the Skills for Health Council. The curriculum, called the "Level 3, 7 Unit Reflexology Practitioners Diploma" consists of 7 pre-defined modules [88]. This modular core curriculum was adopted by all the major accredited reflexology training providers and recognised by CAM/health and beauty vocational awarding bodies, such as City & Guilds, VCTC, ITEC and ABC Awards [88-90]. Reflexology students must meet all the seven module requirements, gain a current first aid certificate and have professional indemnity insurance to be eligible to join the AoR or IFR, although there is no professional obligation to maintain the first aid certification after graduation. BRA membership criteria differs in that they only offer membership to those practitioners who have successfully completed the bespoke Eunice Ingham training at one of the International Institute of Reflexology training centres. However completion of the core curriculum is not a mandatory pre-requisite for professional practice; any person can set up business as a professional reflexologist and operate without professional member or accredited status, regardless of the standard, length or quality of their training.

THE CORE CURRICULUM READING LIST

The Reflexology Forum's core curriculum has a recommended reading list of 29 original teaching texts published on the forum website. When the list was searched for available publications, many of the books appeared be out of print or no longer available, except as second-hand versions. However five of the most popular available teaching texts were still available (excluding the original historical Ingham book). Based on this available sample, the views of the authors of these five books provided a 'snapshot' of what contemporary reflexology educational theorists believe about the appropriateness of reflexology for cardiac patients and what was considered to be the best strategy for treatment of the heart reflex point.

ANALYSIS OF TEACHING TEXTS

The strategy chosen to analyse the responses of each author was to categorise each according to whether their advice constituted a *'therapy specific risk'* belief (implying that reflexology treatment applied to cardiac patients or applied directly to the heart reflex point could have potential adverse/harmful effects) – or like Ingham displayed, a *'no therapy specific risk'* belief (implying that cardiac patient and heart reflex point treatments were considered safe/beneficial). The following five key teaching and theoretic texts were examined using these criteria.

"Reflexology Today" by Doreen Bayley

Bayley was a nurse who studied with Ingham and is generally accredited with bringing Inghams version of reflexology to the UK. She states that reflexology can be of great use in helping various heart conditions; however this recommendation comes with caveats. She advises that the method of treatment should be varied according to the nature of heart trouble, and her claims clearly imply that she believes the heart reflex point to have particularly 'potent' effects on the heart itself. She describes a case where overstimulation of the heart reflex point led to the person having to spend a week in bed recovering. And in the event of a subject (receiver) experiencing a 'heart attack', she states that the therapist should set to work on the heart reflex area found in the left foot as quickly as possible. She states that the impulse effect of this single action has been known to successfully resuscitate many deceased heart attack victims. In cases where the receiver has tachycardia, Bayley also gives a cautionary warning that the therapist should give a general relaxation treatment before approaching the heart reflex point. Her rationale being that if treatment is given to the heart reflex point first, it may adversely increase the elevated pulse rate further. In the case of older subjects with any form of chronic heart disease, Bayley recommends proceeding with caution, advising that the therapist only works for a few minutes on the heart reflex point at first, and only increases the intensity of treatment once the patient has relaxed [91]. Given the caution she advises with regards to treatment of both cardiac patients and the potency she ascribes to the heart reflex point use, it seemed appropriate to categorise Bayley's approach as a 'therapy specific risk' belief in relation to treating cardiac patients and/or the heart reflex point.

"Reflexology: A Better Way to Health" by Nicola Hall

Hall states that the heart reflex point is an important area to work in all cases of heart or circulatory disease [92] and that when any reflex area is worked, there is an increase in the blood circulation to the corresponding organ [93]. More specifically, she claims that reflexology can successfully treat "angina, heart attack, hypertension hypotension…and thrombosis" and for all these conditions, lists the heart reflex point as the key point to work [94]. However she strongly recommends care to be taken when treating the heart reflex area in clients with chronic heart disease due to the risk of "over-stimulating" the heart itself [94]. No clear explanation is given of the over-stimulation process. Based on her cautionary approach to treatment of the heart reflex point in cardiac patients and the potency she ascribes to the heart reflex point use, it seemed appropriate to categorise Hall's approach as a 'therapy specific risk' belief in relation to treating cardiac patients and/or the heart reflex point.

"The Complete Guide to Foot Reflexology" by Kevin and Barbara Kunz

The authors appear to have no concerns about treatment to the heart reflex point or clients with any gradation of cardiac disease. They specifically disregard what they describe as the 'myth' that reflexology can cause a "heart attack", stating that reflexology is "totally safe" [95]. They recommend treating both the heart reflex point and lung area in the event of "heart attacks", along with the sigmoid colon reflex point (in case pocketing of gas has caused the increased pressure on the chest cavity). In cases of angina, they advise treating the heart reflex point "thoroughly". This same confident technique is advised for treating hypertension, except that the solar plexus, kidney and adrenal points are indicated rather than the heart reflex point. Again, the authors stress that reflexologists should work the relevant areas repeatedly and thoroughly to reduce blood pressure. Given that the authors advise no caution when treating cardiac patients and regard reflexology treatment as totally safe for all disease conditions, their approach was categorised as a 'no-therapy specific risk' belief in relation to treating cardiac patients and/or the heart reflex point.

"Reflex Zone Therapy of the Feet: A Textbook for Therapists" by Hanne Marquardt

The author advises caution in treating the heart reflex area and states that it is better to treat the indirect reflex areas rather than the heart point itself. She cites deep vein thrombosis and an aneurysm (if known) as absolute contraindications. For treatment of the heart, the guiding treatment principle is stated as "Depress hyper-excitability and stimulate flaccidity", with "weak stimuli" being seen as beneficial and "strong stimuli" as "detrimental", and "very strong stimuli" as "harmful". The author stresses that this principle of caution, particularly in relation to overstimulation, applies particularly to patients with heart disease [96]. Based on her cautionary approach to treatment of the heart reflex point general and the potency she ascribes to the heart reflex point use, Marquardt's approach was categorised as a 'therapy specific risk' belief in relation to treating cardiac patients and/or the heart reflex point.

"Complete reflexology: Therapeutic Foot Massage for Health and Wellbeing" by Inge Dougans

Although Dougans states that reflexology can do no harm, she advises caution when clients present with thrombosis as she believes treatment could cause the blood clot to move [92]. However she does not offer any cautionary advice regarding treatment techniques to the heart reflex point and there is no indication or contra-indications given in regard to clients with cardiac disease. As the author does not offer any objection to treating cardiac patients and regards reflexology treatment as totally safe for all disease conditions apart from diagnosed thrombosis, her approach was categorised as a 'no-therapy specific risk' belief in relation to treating cardiac patients and/or the heart reflex point.

Given the haemodynamic nature of the core reflexology claim and the continuing importance of these five key teaching texts from the validated recommended reading list, the lack of consensus regarding the appropriateness of reflexology treatment for cardiac patients, particularly in relation to treatment of the heart reflex point itself, was identified as a product safety and quality issue and a significant research challenge. As will be explained shortly, we attempted to address this challenge in our experimental design.

Apart from the variation in teaching content, the other identified product quality issue from contemporary reflexology teaching literature was the variation in published reflexology foot maps. Rather surprisingly, given the central importance of the therapeutic claim of a specific two-way connection between distinct areas of the feet and increased perfusion of the 'mapped' internal organs, the vast majority of published reflexology maps did not appear to exhibit any consensus about where the various reflex points on the feet are. Many different reflexology foot charts were found to be available, ranging from foot maps arbitrarily produced by individual therapists based on their own personal beliefs, right through to maps published and marketed by the Association of Reflexologists [97], the British Reflexology Association [98] and the British School of Reflexology [10]. Most maps appear to have their origins in the original Ingham map [99] but many of the organ-related reflex points on subsequent maps appear in inconsistent places, depending on the beliefs or constructs of the map provider.

This inconsistency of published maps presented a significant research challenge in terms of how to identify the 'correct' heart reflex point location and standardise a treatment strategy for this point.

REDUCTIONIST REFLEXOLOGY TREATMENT

We attempted to overcome the challenge of the inconsistent foot maps and heart reflex point location by developing a novel reductionist reflexology treatment for use as both the active intervention treatment and the control (passive) treatment. With the help of the Association of Reflexologists and the two therapists involved in the study, two forms of treatment were devised for use as the intervention and control. The treatments took account of both the *'therapy specific risk'* belief and *'non-therapy specific risk'* belief by being timed to last just five minutes, with pressure of massage treatment set at 'medium' only. Both consisted of the same number of common, documented reflexology touch techniques, the only difference being that the intervention and control treatments were applied to two different areas of the feet.

As our aim was to isolate the specific effect corresponding with reflexology massage to the heart reflex point area, we proposed a model where reflexology applied to the top part of the foot above Lesfranc's line, served as the 'heart' reflex point area, which made it the active intervention. We believed this strategy to have model validity in terms of the reflexology construct, as the heart reflex point appeared to be consistently placed in the region on either foot above this line. We assumed that if a standardised reproducible set of reflexology therapy massage techniques were applied to this area on both feet, regardless of the imprecise location of the actual heart reflex point, the therapists would, at some point during the treatment to both upper areas, 'hit' or treat the point. Whereas treatment to the feet below the Lefranc's line should result in nothing more than the typical non-specific effects seen with general foot massage, therefore this treatment could act as a passive form of reflexology control. We also believed that this model would overcome the other reflexology research challenge, which is that of establishing an appropriately passive form of control that offers a suitable form of comparison with the active intervention.

Our experiments took the form of a randomised, double-blinded repeated measures trial design, where both the volunteer subjects and data collector were blinded as to the treatment types. During the study, the therapists delivered the active treatment (applied to the upper feet areas) and the passive control treatment (applied to the lower heel area of both feet) to 16 healthy volunteers. All subjects were reflexology-naïve and were allocated to receive either treatment at one of two visits, depending on which treatment they had been assigned to. In order to measure the objective haemodynamic effects of treatment to the heart reflex point, the volunteer subjects were attached to impedance cardiography recording equipment throughout each session (using the Task Force © Monitor). Data was continuously measured from a number of selected cardiovascular data pre, post and intra the treatment sessions. It was hoped that this reductionist treatment design meant all the inherent non-specific effects present in general foot massage would be present in both the intervention and control treatments, allowing any haemodynamic effect on the heart to reveal itself during the 'active' treatment alone. The findings of our experiment revealed an inexplicable cardiovascular effect during the healthy volunteer active treatment sessions. For this group, cardiac index decreased significantly during the left foot 'active' treatment. Furthermore, in this experimental condition, there was a trend towards an increase in total peripheral resistance during the active treatment and a reduction in heart rate when this particular area was being treated, a trend which was not evident in any of the control treatments or when the upper half of the right foot was being treated. Intriguingly, most of the published foot maps, including Ingham's original map, places the heart reflex point somewhere in the left upper foot region. On the basis of these findings, it is tantalising to speculate that our study did reveal a specific haemodynamic effect, as our results suggest that reflexology applied to the upper part of the left foot corresponds with a modest but measurable effect on selected cardiovascular parameters in healthy volunteers. The change in cardiac index indicates that further research is needed to determine if this effect is repeatable in patients with various degree of heart disease and if so, if the effect beneficial or potentially harmful in this patient group.

FUTURE RESEARCH DIRECTIONS

It is clear that there is a lack of data to inform patients, health care providers and funders as to the appropriateness of reflexology therapy in cardiac patients. And a lack of data which makes cost effectiveness analysis possible. However regardless of the significant inconsistencies in its historical narrative and contemporary teaching literature, and the lack of supportive evidence for efficacy [12;100;101], reflexology has gained exceptional worldwide acceptance and is currently used by thousands of healthy people and patients. The use of complementary and alternative therapies in western industrialised countries, even with well-developed conventional health care systems is substantial, ranging from 10-52% [102-104]. There is therefore clearly a public 'need' for these therapies in the general population. Furthermore, complementary therapies including reflexology are increasingly utilised by patients with severe medical conditions and in some areas are offered within conventional health care systems. However, there is insufficient evidence on how this should best integrate with convention health care [105;106] and it seems that when patients use complementary and alternative therapies out with conventional health care services, many do not inform their physician [107;108]. This is a concern if there is potential for interaction, whether for good or bad, between different therapies.

The results of a local survey at our institution indicated that over 9% of patients attending a cardiology clinic purchased reflexology [unpublished data], although its use in patients has been most commonly documented in palliative care [109] and chronic pain [110]. However, cardiac patients are arguably the patients who may have most to gain (or lose) from potential haemodynamic changes (invoked by reflexology) as most cardiac patients have a disease process or drug therapy that specifically alters the body's haemodynamic homeostasis. Although the evidence is lacking in this respect, there does appear to be a high level of patients / client satisfaction with reflexology. However given the lack of robust research in this area, further studies are required to allow the public, patients and healthcare providers to make evidence based decisions on its provision.

CONCLUSION

Modern reflexology reports its roots from zone therapy. However, we have demonstrated that there are significant inconsistencies between the theoretical claims of William H Fitzgerald, Eunice Ingham and key contemporary reflexology educators. Furthermore, while reflexology has gained international popularity, the modern evidence base to confirm or refute the original claims is lacking. Considering its widespread use in the general population and within patient groups, and based on the findings of our healthy volunteer study, there is a clear need for further quality research in this area to help patients, clinicians and healthcare providers make evidence based decision on the role reflexology should have in modern medicine.

REFERENCES

[1]   Mackereth PA, Tiran D. *Clinical Reflexology: A Guide for Health Professionals.* Edinburgh: Churchill Livingstone Elsevier; 2002.

[2]   Ingham E. *Perfect health spells perfect feet. Stories the feet can tell thru reflexology; stories the feet have told thru reflexology.* 11th ed. St Petersburg, Florida: Ingham Publishing; 1984. p. 3-4.

[3]   Hayes J, Cox C. Immediate effects of a five-minute foot massage on patients in critical care. *Complimentary Therapies in Nursing and Midwifery* 2000;6(19):13.

[4]   Hatton J, King L, Griffiths P. The impact of foot massage and guided relaxation following cardiac surgery: a randomised controlled trial. *Journal of Advanced Nursing* 2002;37(2):199-207.

[5]   Bauer BA, Cutshall SM, Wentworth LJ, Engen D, Messner PK, Wood CM, et al. Effect of massage therapy on pain, anxiety, and tension after cardiac surgery: A randomized study. *Complementary Therapies in Clinical Practice 2009*;In Press, Corrected Proof.

[6]   Ejindu A. The effects of foot and facial massage on sleep induction, blood pressure, pulse and respiratory rate: Crossover pilot study. *Complementary Therapies in Clinical Practice* 2007 Nov;13(4):266-75.

[7]   International Institute of Reflexology I. *IIR Diploma Course.* 2012. Ref Type: Online Source.

[8]   IIR IIoR. *Branches of the International Institute of Reflexology.* 2012. Ref Type: Online Source.

[9]   International Institute of Reflexology I. *The nations leading authority.* 2012. Ref Type: Online Source.

[10]   IIR IIoR. *About the IIR.* 2012. Ref Type: Online Source.

[11]   Singh S, Edzard E. *How do you determine the truth?* Reading: Bantam Press; 2008. p. 16-52.

[12]   Ernst E. Is reflexology an effective intervention? A systematic review of randomised controlled trials. *Medical Journal of Australia* 2009;191(5):263-5.

[13]   House of Lords SC. The Individual Disciplines Examined. *House of Lords Select Committee on Science and Technology: Complementary and Alternative Therapies.* 2000. p. 21.

[14] NIFAB NIfab. *NIFAB-undersokelsen.* 2007. Ref Type: Online Source.

[15] ViFAB KaRCfAMIutMotIaH. *Reflexology.* 2005. Ref Type: Online Source.

[16] House of Lords Select Committee H. The Evidence. *House of Lords Select Committee on Science and Technology: Complementary and Alternative Therapies.* HMSO; 2000. p. 45.

[17] Rossana HoF. *Hands on Feet Contact & Prices.* 2010. Ref Type: Online Source

[18] Smallwood C. *The Role of Complementary and Alternative Medicine in the NHS:* An Investigation into the Potential Contribution of Mainstream Complementary Therapies to Healthcare in the UK. FreshMinds; 2010.

[19] Ernst E, Koder K. An overview of reflexology. *European Journal of General Practice* 1997 Jan 1;3(2):52-7.

[20] Robinson N, Lorenc A, Lewith G. Complementary and alternative medicine (CAM) professional practice and safety: A consensus building workshop. *European Journal of Integrative Medicine* 2011;(10):1-6.

[21] Lewith G, Jonas WB, $Walach H. The role of outcomes research in evaluating complementary and alternative medicine. Clinical Research in Complementary Therapies: Principles, Problems and Solutions. *Edinburgh: Churchill Livingstone;* 2002. p. 29-45.

[22] Kiat H, Sun Bin Y, Grant S, Hsu-Tung Chang D. Complementary medicine use in cardiovascular disease: a clinician's viewpoint. *Medical Journal of Australia* 2011;(195):11-2.

[23] Kunz B, Kunz K. *Reflexology.* 1st ed. Dorling Kindersley; 2010.

[24] Ingham E. *Stories the Feet Can Tell Thru Reflexology - Stories the Feet Have Told Thru Reflexology.* Ingham Publishing Inc; 1984.

[25] Bayly D. *Reflexology Today.* 3rd ed. Vermont: Healing Arts Press; 1978.

[26] Marquardt H. *Reflex Zone Therapy of the Feet:* A Textbook for Therapists. 1st ed. Thorsons; 1983.

[27] Dougans I. *Complete Reflexology: Therapeutic Foot Massage for Health and Well-Being.* Bath: Element Books; 1996.

[28] Hall N. *Reflexology for Women.* 1994. London, Thorsons. 4. Ref Type: Online Source

[29] Bisson DA. Reflexology. In: Frishman WH, Weintraub MI, Micozzi MS, editors. Complementary and Integrative Therapies for Cardiovascular Disease. *New York: Elsevier Mosby;* 2005. p. 331-41.

[30] WHO WHO. *World Health Organisation: Traditional Medicine,* Fact sheet no 134. 2012. Ref Type: Online Source

[31] Issel C. *The americans and reflexology. Reflexology; Art, Science & History.* Sacramento, Ca, New Frontier Publishing; 1996. p. 46-81.

[32] Bond Bressler H. Introduction. *Zone Therapy.* 2 ed. Richmond, Virginia: Williams Printing Company; 1971. p. 19-32.

[33] Fitzgerald WH. *Zone Therapy: For Doctors only. Zone therapy or relieving pain at home.* Columbus, Ohio: I W Long Publisher; 1917.

[34] Fitzgerald WH, Bowers EF. Relieving pain by pressure. *Zone Therapy or Relieving Pain at Home.* New York: Kessinger Publishing Co; 1917. p. 15-23.

[35] Fitzgerald WH. Curing Goitre with a probe. *Zone therapy or relieving pain at home.Columbus,* Ohio: I W Long Publisher; 1917. p. 32-41.

[36] Fitzgerald WH. Making the deaf hear. *Zone therapy or relieving pain at home.Columbus,* Ohio: I W Long Publisher; 1917. p. 51-9.

[37] Fitzgerald WH. *Zone therapy for women. Zone therapy or relieving pain at home.* Columbus, Ohio: I W Long Publisher; 1917. p. 76-82.

[38] Fitzgerald WH. Curing Lumbago. *Zone therapy or relieving pain at home.* Columbus, Ohio: I W Long Publisher; 1917. p. 93-103.

[39] Fitzgerald WH. *Scratching hand for sick stomach. Zone therapy or relieving pain at home.* Columbus, Ohio: I W Long Publisher; 1917. p. 104-10.

[40] Fitzgerald WH. *Hay fever, asthma and tonsilits. Zone therapy or relieving pain at home.* Columbus, Ohio: I W Long Publisher; 1917. p. 111-9.

[41] Fitzgerald WH. *That aching head. Zone therapy or relieving pain at home.Columbus,* Ohio: I W Long Publisher; 1917. p. 25-31.

[42] Hall N. *What reflexology is and where it came from. Reflexology for Women.* London: Thorsons; 1994. p. 4-8.

[43] Fitzgerald WH. *Introduction. Zone therapy or relieving pain at home.* Columbus, Ohio: I W Long Publisher; 1917. p. 5-10.

[44] Fitzgerald WH. *Zone therapy - mainly for dentists. Zone therapy or relieving pain at home.* Columbus, Ohio: I W Long Publisher; 1917. p. 148-70.

[45] Fitzgerald WH. *Publishers note. Zone therapy or relieving pain at home.* Columbus, Ohio: I W Long Publisher; 1917. p. 11-2.

[46] Fitzgerald WH, Bowers EF. *Food for thought. Zone Therapy or Relieving Pain at Home.* New York: Kessinger Publishing Co; 1917. p. 186-91.

[47] Connor CD. *Who were the winners in the scientific revolution? A people's history of science; Miners, Midwives and Low Mechanicks.* New York: Nation Books; 2005. p. 404-5.

[48] Beyerstein BL. Alternative medicine and common errors of reasoning. *Academic Medicine* 2001;76(3):230-7.

[49] Ingham E. Preface. *Stories the feet can tell thru reflexology; stories the feet have told thru reflexology.* 11th ed. St Petersburg, Florida: Ingham Publishing; 1984. p. ii-iv.

[50] Ingham E. *Perfect Health Spells Perfect Feet. Stories the Feet Can Tell Thru Reflexology - Stories the Feet Have Told Thru Reflexology.* 1984. p. 3-4.

[51] Ingham E. Zone therapy. *Stories the Feet Can Tell; Stories the Feet Have Told Thru Reflexology.* 4th ed. 1984. p. 6-7.

[52] Ingham E. Reflexes present in the hands and feet. *Stories the feet can tell thru reflexology; stories the feet have told thru reflexology.* 11th ed. St Petersburg, Florida: Ingham Publishing; 1984. p. 10-1.

[53] Ingham E. Location of reflexes. Stories the Feet Can Tell; *Stories the Feet Have Told Thru Reflexology.* 4th ed. 1984. p. 12-3.

[54] Ingham E. *Stories the feet can tell. Stories the feet can tell thru Reflexology; stories the feet have told thru reflexology.* St Petersburg, Florida: Ingham Publishing; 1984. p. 1-2.

[55] Ingham E. Reactions manifested. *Stories the Feet Can Tell; Stories the Feet Have Told Thru Reflexology.* 4th ed. 1984. p. 8-9.

[56] Ingham E. Illustration of technique. Stories the feet have told.St Petersburg, Florida: Ingham Publishing; 1984. p. 12.

[57] International Institute of Reflexology I. IIR Training: *Why settle for less than the best?* 2012. Ref Type: Online Source

[58] Ingham E. *As compared to a watch. Stories the feet can tell thru reflexology; stories the feet have told thru reflexology.* 11th ed. St Petersburg, Florida: Ingham Publishing; 1984. p. 45-6.

[59] Levick J. *Overview of the cardiovascular system. An introduction to cardiovascular physiology.* 5th ed. London: Hodder Arnold; 2010. p. 1-14.

[60] Ingham E. *Introduction. Stories the feet can tell thru reflexology; stories the feet have told thru reflexology.* 11th ed. St Petersburg, Florida: Ingham Publishing; 1984. p. V.

[61] Ingham E. *Gland reflexes in the feet. Stories the feet can tell thru reflexology; stories the feet have told thru reflexology.* 11th ed. St Petersburg, Florida: Ingham Publishing; 1984. p. 6-8.

[62] Ingham E. *Terminals. Stories the feet can tell thru reflexology; stories the feet have told thru reflexology.* 11th ed. St Petersburg, Florida: Ingham Publishing; 1984. p. 67.

[63] Ingham E. *To blaze the path. Stories the feet can tell thru reflexology; stories the feet have told thru reflexology.* 11th ed. St Petersburg, Florida: Ingham Publishing; 1984. p. -93.

[64] Ingham E. *Importance of proper circulation. Stories the feet can tell thru reflexology; stories the feet have told thru reflexology.* 11th ed. St Petersburg, Florida: Ingham Publishing; 1984. p. 104.

[65] Ingham E. Ingham compression method of reflexology. *Stories the Feet Can Tell; Stories the Feet Have Told Thru Reflexology.* 4th ed. 1984. p. 2-3.

[66] Ingham E. *An open mind. Stories the feet can tell thru reflexology; stories the feet have told thru reflexology.* 11th ed. St Petersburg, Florida: Ingham Publishing; 1984. p. 23-4.

[67] Ingham E. *Mind and digestion. Stories the feet can tell thru reflexology; stories the feet have told thru reflexology.* 11th ed. St Petersburg, Florida: Ingham Publishing; 1984. p. 97-9.

[68] Ingham E. *Don't be hasty. Stories the feet can tell thru reflexology; stories the feet have told thru reflexology.* 11th ed. St Petersburg, Florida: Ingham Publishing; 1984. p. 15.

[69] Ingham E. T*he Heart. Stories the feet can tell thru reflexology; Stories the feet have told thru reflexology.* 4 ed. St Petersburg: Ingham Publishing Inc.; 1938. p. 43-8.

[70] Mukherjee D. Complications of Myocardial Infarction. In: Marso S, Griffin BP, Topol EJ, editors. *Cardiovascular Medicine.* London: Lippincott Williams & Wilkins; 2000. p. 39-56.

[71] Jones J, Thomson P, Irvine K, Leslie S. Is there a specific haemodynamic effect in reflexology: A systematic review of randomised controlled trials? *Jouirnal of Alternative and Complementary Medicine.* In press 2011.

[72] Gunnarsdottir JT, Helga J. Does the experimental design capture the effects of complementary therapy? A study using reflexology for patients undergoing coronary artery bypass graft surgery. *Journal of Clinical Nursing* 2007 Apr;16(4):777.

[73] Frankel BSM. The effect of reflexology on baroreceptor reflex sensitivity, blood pressure and sinus arrhythmia. *Complementary Therapies in Medicine* 1997 Jun;5(2):80-4.

[74] Hodgson NA, Andersen S. The Clinical Efficacy of Reflexology in Nursing Home Residents with Dementia. *Journal of Alternative & Complementary Medicine* 2008 Apr;14(3):269-75.

[75] Zhen LP, Fatimah SN, Acharya RU, Tam D-WD, Joseph KP. Study of Heart Rate Variability due to Reflexological Stimulation. *Clinical Accupuncture and Oriental Medicine* 2004;(4):173-8.

[76] Wilkinson ISA, Prigmore S, Rayner CF. A randomised-controlled trail examining the effects of reflexology of patients with chronic obstructive pulmonary disease (COPD). *Complementary Therapies in Clinical Practice* 2006 May;12(2):141-7.

[77] Joseph P, Acharya IR, Kok Poo C, Chee J, Min KC, Iyengar SS, et al. Effect of reflexological stimuylation on heart rate variability. *Innovation et technologie en biologie et medecine* 2004;(25):40-5.

[78] Mackereth PA, Booth K, Hillier VF, Caress AL. Reflexology and progressive muscle relaxation training for people with multiple sclerosis: A crossover trial. *Complementary Therapies in Clinical Practice* 2009 Feb;15(1):14-21.

[79] Mc Vicar AJ, Greenwood CR, Fewell F, D'Arcy V, Chandrasekharan S, Alldridge LC. Evaluation of anxiety, salivary cortisol and melatonin secretion following reflexology treatment: A pilot study in healthy individuals. *Complementary Therapies in Clinical Practice* 2007 Aug;13(3):137-45.

[80] Sudemeier H, Bodner G, Egger I, Mur E, Ulmer H, Herold M. Changes of renal blood flow during organ-associated foot reflexology measured by colour Doppler sonography. *Research in Complementary Medicine: Forschende Komplmentarmedizin* 1999;(5):129-34.

[81] Mur E, Schmidseder S, Egger I, Bodner G, Hartig F, Pfeiffer KP, et al. Influence of Reflex Zone Therapy of the Feet on Intestinal Blood Flow Measured By Color Doppler Sonography. *Forschende Komplementarmedizin und Klassische Naturheilkunde* 2001;(8):86-9.

[82] Black C. *Assessing complementary practice: Building consensus on appropriate research methods.* The King's Fund; 2009.

[83] Stone J. *Development of proposals for a future voluntary regulatory structure for complementary healthcare professions.* The Prince of Wales's Foundation for Integrated Health; 2005.

[84] FWG FWG. *A Federal Approach to Professionally-Led Voluntary Regulation for Complementary Healthcare:* The final report of the Federal Working Group: A plan for action. 2008.

[85] CNHC C&NHC. *Mission and Values.* 2011. Ref Type: Online Source

[86] CNHC C&NHC. *Why register with the Complementary & Natural Healthcare Council.* 2011. Ref Type: Online Source

[87] CNHC C&NHC. *Criteria for Entry to the CNHC Register.* 2011. Ref Type: Online Source

[88] AoR TAoR. *Am I eligible?* 2011. Ref Type: Online Source

[89] The British Reflexology Association B. *What is Reflexology?* 2010. Ref Type: Online Source

[90] IIR TIFoR. *The International Federation of Reflexologists.* 2012. Ref Type: Online Source

[91] Bayley DE. *The Heart. Reflexology Today.* 3rd ed. Rochester: Healing Arts Press; 1982. p. 31-2.

[92] Hall N. *The reflex areas of the feet and hands. Reflexology: A Way to Better Health.* London: Thorsons; 1992. p. 27-91.

[93]   Hall N. *How the treatment works. Reflexology: A Way to Better Health.* Bath: Gateway Books; 1992. p. 115-22.

[94]   Hall N. *The treatment of different disorders. Reflexology: A Way to Better Health.* Bath: Gateway Books; 1992. p. 124-57.

[95]   Kunz K, Kunz B. *You the Reflexologist. The Complete Guide to Foot Reflexology.* London: Thornsons for Harper Collins Publishers; 1984. p. 73-91.

[96]   Marquardt H. *Treatment Procedures. Reflex Zone Therapy of the Feet: A Textbook for Therapists.* 1st ed. Thorsons; 1983. p. 36-65.

[97]   AoR TAoR. *AoR Reflexology Chart.* 2011. Ref Type: Online Source

[98]   BRA BRA. *Reflexology Foot Chart.* 2011. Ref Type: Online Source

[99]   Ingham E. *Stories the Feet Can Tell Thru Reflexology - Stories the Feet Have Told Thru Reflexology.* Ingham Publishing Inc; 1938.

[100] Ernst E, Posadzki P, Lee MS. Reflexology: An update of a systematic review of randomised clinical trials. *Maturitas* 2011 Feb;68(2):116-20.

[101] Wang M, Tsai P, Lee P, Chang W, Yang C. The efficacy of reflexology: systematic review. *Journal of Advanced Nursing* 2008;62(5):512-20.

[102] Eisenberg D, Davis R, Ettner S, Appel S, Wilkey S, Van Rompay M, et al. Trends in alternative medicine use in the United States: Results of a follow-up national survey. *Journal of the American Medical Association* 1998;(280):1569-75.

[103] Metcalfe A, Williams J, McChesney J, Patten S, Jetter N. Use of complementary and alternative medicine by those with a chronic disease and the general population - results of a national population based survey. *BMC Complementary and Alternative Medicine* 2010;(10):58-63.

[104] Thomas K, Coleman P. Use of complementary or alternative medicine in a general population in Great Britain. Results from the National Omnibus survey. *Journal of Public Health* 2004;26(2):152-7.

[105] O'Connor E, White K. Intentions and willingness to use complementary and alternative medicine: what potential patients believe about CAMs. *Complementary Therapies in Clinical Practice* 2009;(15):136-40.

[106] Featherstone C, Godden D, Selvaraj S, Emslie M, Took-Zozaya M. Characteristics assoicated with reported CAM use in patients attending six GP practices in the Tayside and Grampian regions of Scotland: A Survey. *Complementary Therapies in Medicine* 2003;(11):168-76.

[107] Thomson P, Jones J, Evans J, Leslie S. Factors influencing the use of complementary and alternative medicine and wether patients inform their primary care physician. *Complementary Therapies in Medicine.* In press 2011.

[108] Eisenberg DM, Davis RB, Ettner SL, Appel S, Wilkey S, Van Rompay M, et al. Trends in Alternative Medicine Use in the United States, 1990-1997: Results of a Follow-up National Survey. *JAMA* 1998 Nov 11;280(18):1569-75.

[109] Rueda J, Sola I, Pascual A, Subirana CM. *Non-invasive interventions for improving well-being and quality of life in patients with lung cancer. 2011.* Report No.: Cochrane Database Sysetmatic Review CD004282.

[110] van Tulder M, Furlan A, Gagnier J. Complementary and alternative therapies for low back pain. *Best Practice & Research Clinical Rheumatology* 2005;19(4):639-54.

In: Alternative Medicine   ISBN 978-1-62257-106-2
Editors: Kenneth R. Carter and George E. Murphy   ©2012 Nova Science Publishers, Inc.

Chapter 3

PAEDIATRIC ATTENTION-DEFICIT/HYPERACTIVITY DISORDER AND COMPLEMENTARY AND ALTERNATIVE THERAPIES

Fay Karpouzis
Macquarie University, Sydney, Australia

ABSTRACT

According to the systematic reviews the data on the safety, effectiveness and efficacy and long-term use of stimulant medications for paediatric Attention-Deficit/Hyperactivity Disorder (AD/HD) is conflicting. Uncertainty still surrounds the balance of risks and benefits of long-term drug treatment. Current evidence strongly points to significant parental concerns about exposing their children to psychopharmacological interventions. This appears to be the case despite the evidence base for the use of stimulant medications. Children with AD/HD who are treated with stimulants often show side-effects. Across studies, the most frequently examined adverse effects of stimulant medications have been appetite suppression, weight loss, sleep disturbances, irritability, stomach aches, headaches, rashes, nausea, fatigue and occasionally the development or aggravation of tics. Cardiovascular effects and reductions in growth velocity have also been reported. Controversy over the safety and appropriateness of stimulant treatment has led to increased parental anxiety and the increased use of complementary and alternative medicine (CAM) therapies. Many parents prefer to find more natural treatments for their children with AD/HD. In general, parents seek CAM therapies for their children because a particular allopathic treatment was considered ineffective, dissatisfaction with conventional medicine, fear of drug adverse effects and a need for more personal attention for their children. As a result of this controversy, CAM therapies are sought more often by parents who have children with developmental and behavioural disorders such as AD/HD, than with any other condition. The following chapter outlines the variety of CAM therapies available for paediatric AD/HD.

INTRODUCTION

Attention-Deficit/Hyperactivity Disorder (AD/HD) has the distinction of being the most studied and yet most controversial paediatric mental health disorders. [1] It is considered to be the most common disruptive behaviour disorder diagnosed in childhood. [2-5] The American prevalence rates range between 3–7% [2] and 4–12%. [6, 7] The Australian prevalence rates show 11% of 6–17-year-olds are diagnosed with this disorder. [8] The most widely used classification system for mental disorders is the *Diagnostic and Statistical Manual of Mental Disorders, 4th Edition, Text Revision* (DSM-IV-TR). [2, 9-11] The DSM-IV-TR characterises AD/HD as having the essential features of persistent chronic, developmentally inappropriate patterns of "inattention and/or hyperactivity-impulsivity". [2, p.85] Children with AD/HD frequently experience difficulties in academic achievement and behavioural control, finding it difficult to establish positive relationships with family, authority figures and their peers. [3, 4] It has also been shown that AD/HD has long-term adverse effects on academic performance, vocational success, and social-emotional development. [12-16] Given the impairment the symptoms of AD/HD manifest across multiple settings (i.e. home, school, social), much attention has been devoted to the development and evaluation of assessments and treatments for this disorder. [17-20]

Controversy surrounds the treatment choices for this disorder. [12, 21, 22] A plethora of literature has been devoted to the research of AD/HD treatment. [17, 18, 20, 23, 24] The majority of this research appears to be in the area of pharmacological therapies, [17, 18, 25] with less emphasis in psychotherapy and other psychosocial interventions, [26, 27] and even less in the area of complementary or alternative interventions. [28, 29] This may explain why the first line of therapy for children and adolescents with AD/HD is psychopharmacologic. [24, 25, 30-32]

Making a decision as to which treatment intervention to implement for children with AD/HD is as complex as the diagnosis and assessment of this disorder. As AD/HD is a complex disorder, its successful management requires teamwork in order to implement treatment and management strategies to achieve the best results for the child. [17, 23] The American Academy of Child and Adolescent Psychiatry (AACAP) recommend a comprehensive treatment plan taking into account the chronicity and severity of the disorder while reviewing the evidence base for effective therapies (i.e. pharmacological and/or behaviour therapy) as well as considering family choices and parental concerns. [24] The AACAP and the Royal Australasian College of Physicians (RACP) recommend a multidisciplinary care program integrating specialised health professionals, parents, teachers, children and community support services. [24, 33] According to the RACP, the best practice, based on clinical experience and expert opinion, are multimodal treatment strategies. [33] This is where multimodal therapy encompasses combinations of psychopharmacotherapy and psychosocial management strategies (i.e. behaviour therapy, psychoeducation, counselling or support), alongside educational interventions. [33] Although this approach is endorsed by the RACP, [33] the AACAP, [24] and the American Academy of Pediatrics (AAP) [34] as best practice, there is little research that directly addresses the efficacy of this multimodal approach. [33]

The decision to place children or adolescents with AD/HD on psychopharmacological therapies needs to be balanced between the risks of the medications, [26] vurses the detrimental effects the symptoms cause in terms of impairment at school, at home and with peers or authority figures. [17] Numerous clinical trials have demonstrated that pharmacological and psychosocial treatment strategies can either independently or jointly reduce the symptoms and impairments associated with AD/HD. [4, 35-44]

According to Manos and colleagues [45] optimal treatment outcomes can be achieved by appropriate pharmacotherapy combined with psychosocial interventions. Evidence-based treatments for AD/HD include medication management (generally with stimulant medications), behavioural interventions (such as behavioural parent training, school consultation, and direct contingency management), or the combination of pharmacological and behavioural approaches. [31, 46]

The widespread use and evidence for the efficacy of stimulant medications is overwhelming. [24, 25, 30, 32, 39] The National Institute for Health and Clinical Excellence (NICE) guidelines, which were published by the British Psychological Society and The Royal College of Psychiatrists, stated that the single most important recommendation for medication usage as first line treatment was for "severe" AD/HD. [13, 47] The challenge then arises as to what constitutes "severe" AD/HD? The controversial issue that constantly surrounds this disorder has been highlighted once more. Unfortunately, the clinical threshold appears to be socially and culturally influenced and determines whether a particular child is "normal" or not. [48] The question of a suitable threshold for "significant impairments associated with ADHD symptoms" is challenging. [13, p.533] As a result, which children fulfil criteria for "significant impairment" is subject to rater bias, and as such, knowing when to use the NICE guidelines is not straightforward. [13] So, the question of what is "severe" AD/HD is left up to the diagnosing clinician, the parent and/or teacher observations and interpretations of the child's behaviours, making it a subjective opinion of severity.

Despite the recommendation to medicate only "severe" cases, [13] it is estimated that 50%–95% of children with clinically diagnosed AD/HD are medicated with stimulants, [23, 39, 49-54] and, despite this high figure, many still manifest deficits in areas such as learning and organisational skills. As many as 30% of medicated children do not show clinically significant outcomes, and others experience side effects, [25, 38, 39, 50, 52, 55-58] and need to discontinue their medications. [51, 53, 58]

According to many systematic reviews, [22, 26, 59-62] and the Multimodal Treatment Study of AD/HD (MTA) study [44, 63] the data on the safety, effectiveness and efficacy and long-term use of stimulant medications for paediatric AD/HD is conflicting. Uncertainty still surrounds the balance of risks and benefits of long-term drug treatment. [64]

Current evidence strongly points to significant parental concerns about exposing their children to psychopharmacological medications. This is true despite the evidence base for the use of stimulant medications for the treatment of children with AD/HD. [24, 25, 30, 32, 39, 65] Children treated with stimulants, however, often show side effects. [26, 50, 52] Across studies, the most frequently examined adverse effects of stimulant medications were appetite suppression, weight loss, sleep disturbances, irritability, stomach aches, headaches, rashes, nausea, fatigue and occasionally the development or aggravation of tics. [23, 26, 38, 40, 50, 52, 53, 59, 66, 67] Cardiovascular effects and reductions in growth velocity have also been reported. [38, 67, 68]

Despite the fact that psychopharmacological therapies are considered as a need to manage the core biological symptoms of paediatric AD/HD (inattention, hyperactivity, impulsivity and affective aggression), other psychosocial difficulties, such as, aggression, oppositional defiant disorder, conduct disorder, academic underachievement, decreased self esteem, depression, and peer relationship problems still manifest in these children. [31, 39, 53, 69] The consensus statement developed by the National Institute of Health pointed out "stimulant treatments may not "normalize" the entire range of behaviour problems, and children under treatment may still manifest a higher level of some behaviour problems". [14, p. 185] The literature supports this finding, that stimulant medication alone, could not manage all of the problems facing children with AD/HD. [13, 31, 39, 53]

According to Chronis and his colleagues, several limitations of pharmacological treatments highlight the clear need for effective psychosocial treatments to be identified. [39] These limitations include limited effects of stimulant medication on problems such as academic achievement and peer relationships, the fact that up to 30% of children do not show a clear beneficial response to stimulants, the inability to continuously medicate children due to side effects such as insomnia and appetite suppression, the potential adverse long term side effects of taking stimulants, the failure of many adolescents to adhere to medication regimens, and the paucity of evidence supporting long-term beneficial effects of pharmacological therapy on domains of impairment. [39, 70]

Concerns have been highlighted over the side effect profiles of pharmacological therapies. When taking into account the chronic impairment children with AD/HD experience across multiple domains of functioning, multimodal treatments should be considered as a necessity to 'normalise' the behaviour of these children. [39, 52] Parents and teachers are more satisfied when behavioural-psychosocial treatments are added to pharmacotherapy, [21, 71] because there is more compliance among those treated, as well as allowing for a reduction in medication doses thus minimising side effects. [21, 71, 72] Another difficulty found with implementing psychosocial and pharmacologic therapies for AD/HD is the fact that any positive effects gained during the course of the treatment are not maintained with discontinuation of the treatment, and failure to generalise treatments to settings outside the clinical situation. [17, 52] Perhaps these are some of the reasons so many parents seek non-traditional therapies (aka. complementary and alternative medicine [CAM]), in their quest to find other ways to help their children.

NON-TRADITONAL TREATMENTS /COMPLEMENTARY AND ALTERNATIVE MEDICINE THERAPIES FOR AD/HD

The use of complementary and alternative medicine (CAM) has increased over the years in the general population, including children. [73, 74] CAM therapies are sought more often by parents who have children with developmental and behavioural disorders such as AD/HD, than with any other condition. [28, 73, 75, 76] In general, parents seek CAM therapies for their children because a particular treatment was considered ineffective, dissatisfaction with conventional medicine, fear of drug adverse effects and a need for more personal attention. [77, 78]

The National Health Service (NHS) of UK [79] has adopted one of the most commonly used definitions of CAM that is used by the Cochrane Complementary Medicine Field [80]:

Complementary medicine includes all such practices and ideas, which are outside the domain of conventional medicine in several countries and defined by its users as preventing or treating illness, or promoting health and wellbeing. These practices complement mainstream medicine by 1) contributing to a common whole, 2) satisfying a demand not met by conventional practices, and 3) diversifying the conceptual framework of medicine. [80]

The taxonomy of CAM therapies was developed through a consensus process and reflects the diversity of therapies included within the scope of CAM. Acupuncture, aromatherapy, chiropractic, dietary and nutritional therapies, herbal medicine, homeopathy, hypnosis, massage, meditation, osteopathy, and yoga are some of the CAM therapies included in this classification system. [79]

Parents with children diagnosed with AD/HD have a variety of reasons for seeking CAM therapies. [81, 82] Many parents prefer to find more natural treatments for their children with AD/HD. [81, 83] Controversy over the safety and appropriateness of stimulant treatment has led to increased parental anxiety and the increased use of CAM therapies. [28, 77, 84] Major concern regarding the side effect profile of stimulant medications, [65, 73, 77, 82, 83, 85] has been the main reason parents have turned to alternative therapies. [28, 73, 82, 85-88] Other reasons parents seek CAM therapies are due to the chronicity of the disorder, [76] and the fact it affects multiple domains of functioning such as academic, social and behavioural domains. [73]

In 2002, Chan found few systematic studies of the prevalence of CAM use in AD/HD. [28] Estimates of the use of non-traditional treatments (i.e. CAM therapies) varies greatly between 9–46%. [89] In different surveys conducted around the world, CAM use for AD/HD ranged from 12% in Florida, USA; [89] 28% in Israel; [87] 54% in Massachusetts, USA; [84] 64% in Perth, Western Australian; [88] and 67.6% in Melbourne, Australia. [73] In 2007, the US National Health Interview Survey gathered information on CAM use among more than 9,000 children aged 17 and under, finding that approximately 12% of the children had used some type of CAM therapy during the past 12 months, and of those 2.5% used CAM therapies for AD/HD. [90] Figures in surveys vary, as can be seen, and this variance is a function of treatment type, population surveyed (i.e. clinical versus community), time period used (i.e. current versus lifetime use) and geographic location surveyed. [89]

Table 1. Kemper's model of holistic care

Component	Example
Biochemical	Medications, dietary supplements, vitamins, minerals, herbal remedies
Lifestyle	Nutrition; exercise/rest; environmental therapies such as heat, ice, music, vibration, and light; mind-body therapies (behaviour management, meditation, hypnosis, biofeedback, counseling)
Biomechanical	Massage and bodywork, chiropractic and osteopathic adjustments, surgery
Bioenergetic	Acupuncture, radiation therapy, magnets, Reiki, healing touch, qi gong, therapeutic touch, prayer, homeopathy

Source: Task Force on Complementary and Alternative Medicine: Provisional Section on Complementary, Holistic, and Integrative Medicine. [77]

A wide range of CAM therapies are used in children, which can be classified into several categories such as biochemical therapies, lifestyle/mind-body therapies, biomechanical therapies, and bioenergetic therapies. [77] According to Kemper, Table 1 below is just one interpretation of what constitutes holistic care, which also includes CAM therapies.

The biochemical therapies act at the level of biochemistry, with herbal remedies, vitamins and nutritional supplements being the most commonly used. [28, 91-93] Frequently used herbs have been gingko biloba, chamomile, kava kava and valerian, which are thought to aid restlessness, decreased concentration and sleep difficulties associated with AD/HD. [28] Megadose vitamin therapies and mineral supplements (such as iron, pyridoxine, zinc, magnesium, coenzyme Q, along with other supplements, are used in an attempt to treat AD/HD symptomatology. [28]

Mounting evidence suggests that the fatty acid (FA) deficiencies or imbalances may contribute to several common overlapping childhood neurodevelopmental disorders such as AD/HD, dyslexia, dyspraxia (developmental coordination disorder [DCD]), and autistic spectrum disorders (ASD). [94-99] Preliminary evidence from short-term RCTs has shown that supplementing the diet with Omega-3 highly unsaturated fatty acids (HUFA) can alleviate symptoms related to AD/HD, dyslexia and DCD. [96] Clinical and experimental evidence has provided a strong rationale for investigating the use of Omega-3 (ω-3) and/or Omega-6 (ω-6) FAs in the treatment of the behavioural and learning disabilities associated with AD/HD, dyslexia and ASD. [95, 97] Positive results have been found in studies with AD/HD and dyslexia using combinations of ω-3 and ω-6 FAs. [95, 96, 99-101] Although, additional studies are needed to establish the optimal composition of FAs (i.e. ω-3/ω-6 ratio or eicosapentaenoic acid/docosahexaenoic acid ratio) as well as dose–response relationships. [94]

However, not all published trials in the area have demonstrated clear benefits of EFA supplementation for AD/HD symptoms in children. [99, 102-104] So far, the few small studies that have been published on the positive benefits of EFAs for childhood neurodevelopmental disorders, have used different populations (i.e. children with AD/HD, dyslexia, DCD, or ASD), have used different study designs (RCT, open-label trials), different treatments (i.e. ω-3 and/or ω-6 with different combinations/ratios) and have used different outcome measures (i.e. Conners' ADHD Index, Movement Assessment Questionnaire for Children [MABC], Wechsler Objective Reading Dimensions [WORD], Aberrant Behaviour Checklist [ABC], Child Behaviour Checklist [CBCL]) making it difficult to draw conclusive decisions. Given the safety and tolerability of EFAs, [94, 96, 101] and the fact that EFAs are essential for normal brain development and function, [94] large-scale studies are needed to confirm findings of benefits of EFAs for AD/HD in children. [105] Although the current evidence remains mixed, further refinements in study design may be useful in clarifying the effects EFAs have on AD/HD symptomatology. [75] Despite this, EFAs are being considered as an alternative or adjunctive therapy for some children with AD/HD. [100, 106] The authors of a systematic review conducted in 2009 on EFAs and AD/HD concluded that, to date, there is no support for the use of EFA supplements as a primary or supplementary treatment for children with ADHD. [107]

Special mention must be made of the 2005 Oxford-Durham study, by Richardson and Montgomery. [94] A double-blind RCT was designed comparing dietary supplementation of ω-3 and ω-6 fatty acids with placebo for children with dyspraxia (DCD) aged 5–12 years. The study ran for three months and then the placebo group was crossed over to active treatment for an additional three months. Outcomes were assessed at three months and results revealed that no effect of treatment on motor skills was apparent, but significant improvements for active treatment versus placebo were found in reading, spelling, and behaviour. After the crossover, similar changes were seen in the placebo-active group, whereas children continuing with active treatment maintained or improved their progress. [94] This study was a very well designed study, meeting the CONSORT recommendations for reporting of RCTs, as all items in the checklist were met. The published article discussed the study design and the rationale for using the type of placebo and time frame; the eligibility criteria for the participants were well explained; the recruitment process, the settings and the data collection locations were described; precise detail of the intervention for each group and how many and when and where they were administered was discussed as well as measures to assess compliance; randomisation, allocation and concealment were all detailed; the outcomes were established prior to commencement of study; the power calculations were explained and the justification for the figures was outlined; followed by the explanation for the statistical analyses and rationale for undertaking such analyses.

The results from Oxford-Durham study also followed the CONSORT recommendations by starting with the flow diagram showing the flow of participants through the study and indicating numbers eligible, excluded, non-compliant and completing study with appropriate outcome measures. The results included tables of the three outcome measures and all the data collected at baseline, months 3 and 6 with the statistical analyses.

The conclusions drawn from the Oxford-Durham study were that although no effect of treatment on motor skills was evident, improvements in literacy skills and behaviour found were consistent with other reports of benefits from fatty acid supplementation among children with dyslexia or ADHD. [99, 106] The authors indicated that the "similarity in the effect sizes for ADHD-related symptoms" between the DCD sample and dyslexia and AD/HD samples could suggest that the results may be more widely generalisable. [94, p.1365]

Furthermore, despite the fact the Oxford-Durham study focused on DCD, the authors suggest that approaching the neurodevelopmental disorders via a symptom-based approach could be more productive and more beneficial for children, as there is such high comorbidity and symptom overlap between DCD, AD/HD, dyslexia and ASD. [94] This study was mentioned for two reasons. First, others have also suggested that children with these overlapping neurodevelopmental disorders may be better served if focus shifted from labelling them with diagnostic categories to dealing with the symptoms. [108]

There is growing concern that the DSM diagnostic categories do not reflect the way in which the neurodevelopmental disorders affect real people. [109] Furman hypothesised that "AD/HD is not a distinct neurologic or psychological disease entity", but instead "might represent a final common behavioural pathway for a gamut of emotional, psychological, and/or learning problems". [108, p.998] This idea concurs with the "symptom-based approach" that the Oxford-Durham study researchers proposed as a result of their findings. [94]

Secondly, if CAM researchers and CAM practitioners want CAM therapies to be considered as a possible option for the treatment and management of paediatric AD/HD then CAM therapies must undergo scientific scrutiny. Unfortunately, most CAM therapies still await proper scientific evaluation. [110] Perhaps if researchers of CAM therapies conducted RCTs with high quality methodological practices such as those outlined by the CONSORT group, then perhaps the results will have a higher probability of being reliable and valid, such as those in the Oxford-Durham study.

Lifestyle/Mind-body interventions are therapies that can be included in the daily lives of children with AD/HD, such as nutrition, exercise, environmental changes; and mind-body techniques such as psychotherapy (including CBT), hypnosis and biofeedback. [28] Lifestyle/Mind-body therapies are geared toward utilising the mind's ability to influence the body's functions and symptoms. For children with AD/HD, the mind-body therapies are designed to help decrease autonomic hyperarousal to stress by evoking a relaxation response. There are a variety of techniques for relaxation training such as, meditation, muscle relaxation, deep breathing, hypnosis, and biofeedback. All of these are designed to educate the child with AD/HD to relax, and therefore create a decrease in their autonomic activity. [28]

The most popular alternative therapy for AD/HD has been dietary manipulation. [17, 23, 28, 53, 75, 83, 87, 88, 92] The major dietary interventions for AD/HD that have emerged over the last century have been the Feingold and Feingold-like diets, the low-sugar or sugar elimination diets and the oliogoallergenic/oligoantigenic ("few foods") diet. [75] The surveys conducted in Australia, Israel and the USA regarding AD/HD and CAM use all included dietary modifications, [73, 84, 87-89] with findings that dietary manipulations were the most frequently used alternative therapy. [73, 87, 88] In contrast to this, a study conducted in a developmental medical centre in Australia found less than one third of the sample had tried dietary manipulation, with the expressive therapies (e.g. music, dance, sensory integration, and occupational therapy) being more common. [84] A study conducted in a developmental referral centre in Western Australia, found that dietary manipulation was the most frequently explored alternative therapy with 60% of children diagnosed with AD/HD having used Feingold-like diets, sugar restrictions, allergy-based diets, multivitamins, and naturopathic supplementation. [88] Another interesting finding from this study is that there was no statistical difference in the prevalence use of CAM therapies between medicated and non-medicated children with AD/HD. [88] This implies that many parents are willing try CAM therapies for their children regardless of whether they opt for medications or not. In a study conducted in the Royal Children's Hospital in Melbourne Australia, 66% of those surveyed had used dietary manipulation for their children diagnosed with AD/HD. [73] In a survey conducted in the Neuropaediatric Unit in Shaare Zedek, Israel, the most common CAM modality used was also dietary intervention with 14.4% of those surveyed. [87]

Although much research has been conducted in the area of dietary interventions, the scientific merit of the published studies is varied. [75] In 1975, Feingold reported behavioural improvement in 50% of children with AD/HD when foods were eliminated from their diet if they contained natural or artificial salicylates. [111] A meta-analysis [112] and several systematic reviews [113-115] concluded that the Feingold diet was not effective for hyperactive behaviours. Methodological flaws such as poor definition of sample, not specifying consistent diet, not using appropriate placebos or controls, not using adequate dose of artificial additives or colourings, and not describing outcome measures in a standardised manner were cited as the reasons for these negative conclusions. [75] According to the NICE guidelines, the quality of the evidence for dietary interventions is generally poor, reflecting the paucity of the data and the evidence is inconclusive that elimination or supplementation diets, when compared with placebo, may reduce AD/HD symptoms. [13] However, the NICE guidelines do recommend and recognise the value of a balanced diet, good nutrition and regular exercise for children and young people with AD/HD. Furthermore, they recommend a food diary for parents with children who have AD/HD. If a link between the child's diet and behaviour is discovered then healthcare professionals are advised to refer parents to a dietician so they can design a specific dietary elimination plan for the child. [13]

The Western Australian Pregnancy Birth Cohort (Raine study) is an ongoing longitudinal study following 2,868 children from utero to 17 years of age. [68] Within the Raine cohort there is a subgroup of children diagnosed with AD/HD. A comparison of the medicated vurses the non-medicated AD/HD subgroup found that there was a "lack of significant improvements in long-term social, emotional and academic functioning associated with the use of stimulant medication". [68, p.7] The results also indicated that between the age of 8 and 14 years there was an average elevation 10mmHg on diastolic blood pressure with stimulant medication usage. [68]

Furthermore, whilst investigating the dietary patterns in the Raine population-based study, it was found that the Western-style diet may be associated with AD/HD. [116] A higher score for a Western-style dietary pattern was associated with the odds (odds ratio = 2.21, 95% confidence interval = 1.18, 4.13) of having an AD/HD diagnosis in adolescents at age 14. When examining the intake of major specific foods that contributed to the Western-style dietary pattern: takeaway foods, processed meats, high-fat dairy products, and soft drinks, were associated with an AD/HD diagnosis. The 'healthy' dietary pattern was not associated with AD/HD, where 'healthy' diet included high intakes of whole grains, fruit, vegetables, legumes and fish. [117] This is the "first study to link a Western style diet with clinical diagnoses for AD/HD and is, therefore, of great interest and importance". [116, p. 407]

Biofeedback techniques studied for children with AD/HD are the electromyogram (EMG) biofeedback and the electroencephalogram (EEG) biofeedback. [28, 92] Electromyogram (EMG) biofeedback is a technique that helps a child develop awareness of muscle tension and it teaches them how to reduce it, resulting in relaxation. [28] Electroencephalogram (EEG) biofeedback's function is to train the patient to self-regulate their brainwave patterns in order to increase concentration, improve mood or reduce distraction, impulsivity and dependency. [83] In 2005, a review by Monastra and colleagues found EEG biofeedback was "probably efficacious" for the treatment of AD/HD with significant clinical improvement reported in 75% of studies. [118, p.95]

During the past three decades, a series of case and controlled group studies examining the effects of EEG biofeedback have reported improved attention and behavioural control, increased cortical activation on quantitative electroencephalographic examination, and gains on tests of intelligence and academic achievement in response to EEG treatment. [118] A review of records was carried out in a private educational setting in 1998 by Thompson and Thompson to examine the results obtained when students with Attention Deficit Disorder (ADD) received 40 sessions of training that combined neurofeedback with the teaching of metacognitive strategies. Because this study was not a controlled scientific study, the efficacious treatment components could not be determined. Regardless, the positive outcomes of decreased ADD symptoms plus improved academic and intellectual functioning suggested that the use of neurofeedback plus training in metacognitive strategies was a useful combined intervention for students with ADD. [119]

Bioenergetic therapies are purpoted to restore the harmonious balance of an invisible energy or spirit that surrounds and flows through the body. The most common forms of these therapies include: acupuncture, therapeutic touch, prayer and homeopathy. Studies in AD/HD and acupuncture are being conducted as acupuncture enters the realm of conventional medicine. [28]

Therapeutic touch is believed to transfer so-called healing energy between the therapist and the patient, in order to release energy blockages within the patient's energy flow. The therapist does not make contact with the patient's body, but instead works with the so-called invisible energy fields surrounding the patient's body. Other therapies that work on a similar principle are Qi Gong, Healing Touch and Reiki. [28]

Homeopathic therapy relies on two principles; that like cures like, and the more dilute the remedy, the more potent it is. [75, 120] There has been increased interest in homeopathy's potential as a non-pharmacological intervention for AD/HD as an alternative to the use of stimulant medications such as Ritalin. [121, 122] There have been mixed results regarding the effectiveness of homeopathy for children with AD/HD. A randomised, double-blind, placebo-controlled crossover trial for homeopathic treatment of children with AD/HD was conducted by Frei and colleagues in 2005. [120] The trial suggested that scientific evidence exists for the effectiveness of homeopathy in the treatment of AD/HD, particularly in the areas of behavioural and cognitive functions. [120] Three other clinical trials also reported improvements for homeopathic therapy for AD/HD in parent ratings of behaviour on both nonstandard [123] and standardised rating scales [120, 124] Contrary to these findings, a study conducted in the same year by Jacobs and colleagues found no evidence to support a therapeutic effect of individually selected homeopathic remedies in children with AD/HD. [125] A review to assess the safety and effectiveness of homeopathy as a treatment for AD/HD was conducted for the Cochrane Database of Systematic Reviews. [121, 122] Data from four eligible studies (total n = 168) were extracted and analysed. To date, the results found that the homeopathic therapies evaluated did not suggest significant treatment effects for the global symptoms, core symptoms of inattention, hyperactivity or impulsivity, or related outcomes such as anxiety in AD/HD. As a result of this review, the current findings point to the existence of little evidence for the efficacy of homeopathy for the treatment of AD/HD. [121, 122, 125]

The biomechanical therapies involve treatments such as chiropractic and massage. However, there are few studies evaluating their effectiveness in treating children with AD/HD. [28, 126] It is believed that massage is used to increase blood flow, which in turn increases the circulating endorphins promoting relaxation and decreasing stress levels. A study by Field and colleagues showed massage therapy to decrease fidgeting and improve scores on the Conners' Scale in adolescents with AD/HD. [127] Fields has hypothesised that massage therapy increases serotonin levels, [128] and as a result of this it may modulate elevated levels of dopamine in children with AD/HD. [129] A pilot study was conducted to examine whether massage or exercise therapy would be effective in reducing symptoms or medication dose in AD/HD combined subtype school age children already stabilised on medication and/or behavioural modification. [129] Both the massage and exercise therapy interventions took place with parents attending. Parents watched the interventions and were instructed on how to perform the massage or help with the exercises at home. A qualitative analysis revealed that all parents involved in the study indicated a positive experience for them and their children. The Conners' Rating Scale indicated an improvement for children in the massage therapy group, according to the parent but not the teacher rating scales. Positive comments reported after 6 weeks in the massage group were better, with improved anger control, improvement in mood, more restful sleep and an improvement in social functioning, and improvement in focusing at school. In the exercise group it was reported that there was improvement in the ability to do homework and to cope in stressful situations. The objectives of this project were difficult to comment on due to the small sample size, and thus clinically significant data were not available; however, the experience of both the children and the families was positive. Although there were no statistical analyses conducted, a trend of improved symptomatology was evident within the massage therapy group. The researcher acknowledges that research in this area is lacking and the encouraging results of this pilot study can lead further to research in this area. [129]

Chiropractic is a leading system of natural healthcare and is practiced worldwide. The World Health Organization, [130] defines chiropractic as:

> ...healthcare profession concerned with the diagnosis, treatment and prevention of disorders of the neuromusculoskeletal system and the effects of these disorders on general health. There is an emphasis on manual techniques, including joint adjustment and/or manipulation ... [130, p.3]

According to the World Federation of Chiropractic (WFC), chiropractors consider themselves to be the "the spinal health care experts in the health care system". [131] Chiropractors are providers of spinal manipulation, spinal adjustments and other manual treatments, exercise instruction and patient education on wellness and lifestyle changes. Chiropractic places great emphasis on the relationship between the spine and the nervous system by improving the function of the neuromusculoskeletal system. With this approach, chiropractors believe they improve overall health, wellbeing and quality of life of their patients. The focus of chiropractic is a patient-centred approach encompassing the principles of the biopsychosocial model of health care. The biopsychosocial principles were formally adopted by the WFC in 2005 and highlight the relationship between the mind and the body in health, the power of the individual to self-heal, the responsibility of each individual for their health while promoting patient autonomy. [131]

Newer forms of chiropractic are expanding to incorporate biopsychosocial approach for the treatment and management of patients, such as the Neuro Emotional Technique (NET). It has been stated that over 100 different chiropractic techniques exist. [132] As early as 1910, DD Palmer, the "father" of chiropractic recognised the importance of "trauma, toxicity and autosuggestion" the so-called "triad of health" in health and disease. [133] Chiropractic has based its practices on DD Palmer's philosophy that health and wellbeing is a balance between physical, mental and chemical factors. However, over the years, chiropractors have focused primarily on the physical aspects of this triad, as the chiropractic profession gained its recognition as musculoskeletal practitioners. The triad of health has gained acceptance once again, as it is in alignment with the biopsychosocial principles outlined by the profession's governing body, the WFC, [131] and the WHO guidelines, [130] and has been adopted within the scope of chiropractic practice.

The American Academy of Pediatrics recognised the increasing use of CAM therapies in children and, as a result, assembled a Task Force on Complementary and Alternative Medicine in 2008 to address issues related to the use of CAM for this population. [77] This task force found that chiropractic care is one of the most common CAM practices provided at the professional level. [77] Recent studies have confirmed that up to 14% of all chiropractic visits were for paediatric patients, [76, 134] and that chiropractors were the most common CAM providers visited by children and adolescents. [77, 134] Studies indicate that adult populations seek chiropractic care predominantly for musculoskeletal complaints. [135] In contrast, paediatric populations seek chiropractic care predominantly for non-musculoskeletal conditions or when asymptomatic. [136]

A survey conducted in the USA on the presenting complaints of paediatric (under 18 years of age with a mean age of 6.9 years) patients for chiropractic care found that parents consulted chiropractors for their children's musculoskeletal (MSK) and non-musculoskeletal (non-MSK) conditions in addition to wellness care. [136] Of these paediatric chiropractic visits, 44% were for MSK conditions and the rest were for non-MSK conditions. [136] Typical MSK conditions treated/managed by chiropractors in a paediatric population were torticollis, neck pain and low back pain, headaches, hip, shoulder and extremity complaints. [136] The most common non-MSK conditions parents seek chiropractic care for their children were asthma, enuresis, colic, ear infections, immune dysfunction, constipation, acid reflux and hyperactivity, to name a few. [136] The same survey also found that the majority of parents who consulted chiropractors for their children's complaints were more likely to be educated at the tertiary level (40% bachelor's degree; 21% college education; 12% master's degree; and 4% doctoral degree). [136]

A survey conducted in Australia of paediatric chiropractic care for children under 18 years of age found that parents (like their American counterparts) also seek care from chiropractors for both MSK and non-MSK complaints. [137] The types of disorders parents seek care for their children differed by age group, but overall the types of MSK conditions presented were headaches, lower back pain, scoliosis and postural problems. The types of non-MSK presenting complaints bought to the attention of chiropractors were: sleeping problems, teething problems, gastric reflux, asthma, irritability, behavioural problems, AD/HD, learning difficulties, nocturnal enuresis, ear infections, upper respiratory tract problems, fatigue and gastro-intestinal problems. [137]

The Neuro Emotional Technique (NET), which is one of the top fifteen techniques used by chiropractors in Australasia and North America, [138] embraces the biopsychosocial principles that are promoted by the WFC and the WHO organisations. Walker designed a therapeutic intervention called NET for MSK and non-MSK conditions with these principles in mind. [139] An analysis of self-reported symptoms from new adult patients presenting to a multi-chiropractor NET clinic, found that the scope of NET patients and their presenting complaints had a higher degree of non-MSK conditions than that usually reported in non-NET chiropractic offices. [140] In this survey, 54.8% (417/761) of the primary complaints were of a MSK nature and 36.0% (274/761) of the primary complaints were of a non-MSK nature, and the other 9.2% presented for maintenance care. [140] The types of non-MSK complaints outlined were immune and recurrent infections (13.9%), stress and anxiety (12.5%), depression (10.9%), fatigue and lethargy (10.2%), female reproductive conditions (7.3%), digestive problems (7.3%), skin and eye disorders (6.9%), attentional difficulties (3.6%), eating disorders (3.6%), insomnia (3.3%), migraine (2.9%) other (8.4%) and 9.2% patients reported they had no primary complaint. The NET clinics are not typical of chiropractic clinics and NET therapy does not fit the traditional mechanistic models proposed by many chiropractors. A survey of NET practitioners investigating paediatric complaints is needed in order to discover whether similar patterns of use exist among the paediatric population.

In 2007, a systematic review was conducted to evaluate the evidence on the effect of chiropractic care on patients with non-MSK conditions. [141] The results found 179 papers addressing 50 different non-MSK conditions. Of these, 122 were case reports or case series, 47 were experimental designs (including 14 RCTs), nine systematic reviews and one was a large cohort study. The 14 RCTs addressed ten different non-MSK conditions. The RCTs were evaluated using the Scottish Intercollegiate Guidelines Network (SIGN) and Jadad checklists; a checklist developed from the CONSORT guidelines; and one developed by the authors to evaluate studies in terms of Whole Systems Research (WSR) considerations. [141] The authors rated the RCTs and found that six RCTs were rated "high" on three checklists (SIGN, Jadad, CONSORT); one of these was also rated "high" in terms of WSR considerations. The conditions that were addressed for chiropractic care using RCT designs were: asthma (n = 3); hypertension (n = 2); dysmenorrhoea/PMS (n = 1); infantile colic (n = 2); otitis media (n = 1); nocturnal enuresis (n = 1); pneumonia (n = 1); phobia (n = 1); and jet lag (n = 1) where 'n' denotes the number of studies. The author's conclusions were that evidence from controlled studies and usual practice supports chiropractic care (the entire clinical encounter) as providing benefit to patients with asthma, cervicogenic vertigo, and infantile colic. Evidence was also promising for potential benefit of manual procedures for children with otitis media and elderly patients with pneumonia. [141] This review also found that the majority of studies conducted for chiropractic care and AD/HD and/or learning disabilities were of case series (n = 4), a case report (n = 1) and a uncontrolled, non-random single subject design study (n = 1) (where 'n' denotes the number of studies). [141] It was noted that adverse effects were not routinely reported and recommendations were made to change this in future research projects. However, the few studies that did report on adverse effects of spinal manipulation for all ages and conditions found that they were rare, transient, and non-severe occurrences. [141]

It is obvious that the parents seek chiropractic care for their children's AD/HD, attentional, behavioural and learning disabilities from chiropractors, both in Australia [137] and the US. [136] The efficacy of treatment for non-musculoskeletal disorders in the paediatric and adolescent chiropractic populations is under-researched. Few RCTs have demonstrated significant clinical benefits of chiropractic practices among paediatric patients. [141] For this reason it is important to conducted high quality methodological sound research projects in an area gaining popularity in a vulnerable population without the evidence to support its practices.

A systematic review of the chiropractic literature was conducted in order to evaluate the evidence of the effect of chiropractic care for the treatment and/or management of children and adolescents with AD/HD. [142] According to this systematic review 15 case studies have been published [143-157]; three case series [158-160]; one single subject design study (n=7) [161]; two uncontrolled, non-random experimental trials (n=41 and n=13) [162, 163]; and one controlled, non-random, experimental clinical trial (n=24) [164] for AD/HD and chiropractic care. Of these, two studies targeted adult AD/HD populations [158, 162], three studies targeted paediatric and adolescent populations [161, 163, 164]. It was obvious from this review that there is a paucity of studies on paediatric and adolescent AD/HD and that the most predominant type of research design is the case study. The methodological quality overall was poor and none of the studies qualified using inclusion criteria. [142]

As a result, the findings of this 2010 systematic review have been classified as an 'empty review'. [142] No high quality evidence was found to evaluate the efficacy of chiropractic care for paediatric and adolescent AD/HD. The claims made by chiropractors that chiropractic care improves AD/HD symptomatology for children and adolescents is only supported by low levels of scientific evidence (i.e. Levels III and IV). [142] The authors concluded that in the interest of paediatric and adolescent health, if chiropractic care is to continue for this clinical population, more rigorous scientific research needs to be undertaken to examine the efficacy and effectiveness of chiropractic treatment for AD/HD. Adequately-sized RCTs using clinically relevant outcomes and standardised measures to examine the effectiveness of chiropractic care verses no-treatment/placebo (control) or standard care (pharmacological and psychosocial care) are needed to determine whether chiropractic care is an effective alternative or adjuvant intervention for paediatric and adolescent AD/HD. [142]

One such study was conducted investigating a technique used by some chiropractors called NET for paediatric AD/HD. [165] This study was an approved clinical trial which was conducted in four private clinics in Sydney, Australia and the protocol has been published in detail elsewhere. [166] Children aged 5-12 years who met inclusion criteria were randomised into three groups: Group A (Sham n = 37), Group B (NET therapy n = 59) and Group C (Control [usual care] n = 32). All groups continued with their existing treatment regimens (i.e. pharmacological and/or psychosocial). Groups A and B had sham and NET protocols added respectively to existing regimens. Psychometric outcome measures were chosen from the Conners' Rating Scales (CRS), which were scored and interpreted by independent registered clinical psychologists. The psychologists, participants, parents and teachers of groups A and B were all blinded to group allocation of the children. An analysis of covariance was conducted comparing the changes between baseline and final results (i.e. after seven months and 14 interventions) between the active group (NET) and placebo group (sham). [165]

The results showed that forty-one participants (10 sham; 21 NET; 10 Control) completed the protocol. According to Conners, the CRS classified changes of five or more subscale points as significant and thus -5 was chosen as the minimally clinically important difference (MCID) for this study. Decreases in global and behavioral indices were indicative of improvements in participants' behaviors and were considered clinically meaningful results. At the conclusion of the study, only

the NET therapy group achieved the MCID ($\geq$-5). The intention to treat analysis revealed that NET therapy produced significant results for all primary and secondary outcomes: Conners' ADHD Index (p = 0.000, CI: -13.03, -3.96); Conners' Global Index (p = 0.006, CI: -13.70, -2.46); DSM-IV:Inattentive (p = 0.031, CI: -9.94, -0.49); DSM-IV:Hyperactive/Impulsive (p = 0.003, CI: -13.91, -2.98) and DSM-IV:Total (p = 0.006, CI: -12.75, -2.23). The Cohen's d coefficient revealed medium to high effect sizes (1.08, 0.82, 0.64, 0.89 and 0.82, respectively). These significant results denote improvements in global and behavioral indices (i.e. reductions in inattention, hyperactivity and impulsivity) in participants who received NET therapy in addition to usual care. [165]

The authors concluded that these results provided the first data towards answering the question: "Does NET have a potential role to play in the management of pediatric AD/HD?" This study demonstrated clinically meaningful changes and significant results for the emotional component of NET therapy for pediatric AD/HD. However, definitive recommendations could not be made about the intervention at the time until a protocol using the whole spectrum of NET is undertaken. [165]

INTEGRATIVE APPROACHES TO AD/HD

Integrative medicine provides care that is patient centred, healing oriented, emphasises the therapeutic relationship, and uses therapeutic approaches originating from conventional and alternative medicine. [77, 167] The integrative practitioner actively seeks to avoid risky and unproven pharmacological interventions if possible. [168] The integrative practitioner focuses more on symptom patterns than on DSM diagnosis. A whole-child approach naturally de-emphasises labels and limitations of the current diagnostic system. [168] The last two decades have seen a dramatic rise in the number of children given psychiatric medications. If current rates persist, within a generation, half of American children will be taking psychiatric medication. [168] This should concern all of us, as parents, practitioners, the public and the policymakers should be endeavouring to work together to change this trend.

A review conducted by Kidd has led to the suggestion that an integrative approach produces the best results for children with AD/HD. [169] Kidd believes that AD/HD has become a "testing ground for modern holistic/integrative medical management", as an alternative to the "mainstream" choice of prescription stimulants. [169, p.420] According to Kidd, safe and more effective treatment options are readily available for children with AD/HD. Firstly, Kidd advises dietary interventions for AD/HD symptomatology as the benefits of the nutrients are broader in their spectrum of positive effects and have a superior benefit-to-risk profile than medications. [169] The removal of food additives, sensitising foods, and sugar (sucrose), followed by an assessment for allergies, nutrient deficiencies, and intolerances to foods and chemicals, is highly recommended by Kidd. Following that, an assessment and correction of any toxic burdens to the body, including lowering of potentially toxic metals (e.g. lead) should be addressed. Kidd believes that by using dietary supplementation practitioners may still prescribe medications, as nutrients are far more compatible with drugs than the compatibility of drugs with other drugs. [169]

Harding and colleagues conducted a pilot study to compare Ritalin® (the stimulant Methylphenidate) and food supplements. [170] Outcomes were compared using the Intermediate Visual and Auditory/Continuous Performance Test (IVA/CPT) and the two-way analysis of variance with repeated measures and with Tukey multiple comparisons. [170] Harding and colleagues found the extensive literature review by Kidd, [169] strongly supported a heterogeneous molecular aetiology for AD/HD. [170] Using Kidd's review and other published studies they found the biochemical heterogeneous aetiologies for AD/HD cluster around at least eight risk factors: food and additive allergies, heavy metal toxicity and other environmental toxins, low-protein/high-carbohydrate diets, mineral imbalances, essential fatty acid and phospholipid deficiencies, amino acid deficiencies, thyroid disorders, and B-vitamin deficiencies. [170]

The dietary supplements used for the pilot study were a mix of vitamins, minerals, phytonutrients, amino acids, essential fatty acids, phospholipids, and probiotics that attempted to address the AD/HD biochemical risk factors. The results revealed that participants in both groups showed significant gains (p< 0.01) on the IVA/CPT, Full Scale Response Control Quotient and Full Scale Attention Control Quotient (p<0.001). Their findings support the effectiveness of food supplement treatment in improving attention and self-control in children with AD/HD and suggest food supplement treatment of AD/HD may be of equal efficacy to

Ritalin treatment. [170] However, the authors/researchers recognised that this was only a pilot study with n = 20 and that further research is needed in this area. [170]

There is very little published in the area of AD/HD and integrative medicine. However, if the two fields of health care (i.e. conventional western medicine and CAM) could come together under the banner of integrative medicine, greater benefits can be imparted to the children suffering from the symptoms of AD/HD. With the two disciplines working together then perhaps a variety of safe and effective evidence-based alternatives for children can be offered from the CAM practitioners while the conventional practitioners can work to slowly reduce medications until they are no longer needed. If practitioners are willing to embrace the biopsychosocial principles and integrate therapies such as nutraceuticals (vitamin and mineral supplements), nutrition, exercise, massage, chiropractic, biofeedback, behaviour management, family therapy and educational interventions to name a few, then collectively the team increases the probability of meeting all of the health needs of a particular patient.

CAM CONCLUSIONS

Generally speaking, most parents who have tried at least one CAM therapy for their children with AD/HD find it helpful. [73] The finding that modified diet was the commonest therapy tried is in keeping with many previous studies, [73] with chiropractic care being the most popular CAM therapy for the paediatric population. [77, 134] The CONSORT group who assessed the quality of systematic reviews conducted for CAM therapies for paediatric populations found that the commonest CAM therapy used was vitamin therapy. [171] The initial evidence for some CAM therapies such as dietary modifications, essential fatty acid supplementation, biofeedback, yoga, massage, homeopathy and green outdoor spaces suggest potential benefits as part of or as an overall treatment plan for AD/HD. [75] Much of the CAM therapy research suffers from methodological weaknesses, such as lack of large sample sizes, lack of blinding, lack of control groups, lack of random assignment between active treatment and control/placebo groups, and lack of standardised outcome measures to name just a few, [128] which makes it no different from research conducted in conventional medical trials.

In 2002, the CONSORT group assessed the quality of randomised trials for CAM therapies within the paediatric population as a result of the increase usage of CAM for this population. At that time, only 40% of the CONSORT checklist items were included in the published articles. [171] Recommendations made at that time were for CAM researchers to conduct and report CAM trials with the highest possible standards in order for these types of studies to become a valid source of information for the paediatric population. [171]

The increase use of CAM therapies for children (under 18 years) has seen an increase of publications in RCTs for paediatric complementary and alternative medicine in the literature since 1965. [172] It is interesting to note that the reports of the RCTs of CAM therapies for this population are published in 'mainstream' medical journals (such as The American Journal of Clinical Nutrition, Pediatrics, Journal of Pediatrics, and Lancet) and not in alternative journals. [172] In fact, of the 908 RCTs sourced for one review for paediatric CAM therapies, 93% were Medline indexed. [172] An evaluation conducted by the Task Force on Complementary and Alternative Medicine found that the quality of RCTs of CAM was as good as that of RCTs of conventional medicine. [173] Furthermore, this task force found that the quality of systematic reviews of CAM exceeded that of systematic reviews of conventional medicine. [174]

The fact that CAM RCTs are being published in mainstream journals is a positive finding indicating that CAM is not only gaining acceptance within the public arena but also the medical arena. Overall, the future of CAM therapies is promising; however, more high quality methodologically sound research in the format of double-blind controlled clinical trials, systematic reviews and meta-analyses are required to determine what place CAM therapies have in the treatment and management of paediatric and adolescent AD/HD.

SUMMATION

From the vast amount of literature written on the subject of AD/HD, it is evident that this common condition is extremely complex in nature, and many questions still exist about its treatment and management. Even though treatment and management has been seen to be multidisciplinary, requiring the collaboration of mental health, educational, and medical professionals, the focus has largely been on pharmacological treatments. The majority of research in psychopharmacology has been focused on stimulants, with varied outcomes in terms of safety and efficacy, and yet there have been dramatic increases in its use over the past two decades. Considering there appears to be much debate and conflict regarding the safety and efficacy of current pharmacological treatments for AD/HD among children, researchers have been examining other modes of therapy. Research findings also show evidence for psychosocial therapies and combined therapies (i.e. psychosocial and pharmacological therapies) for the treatment and management of paediatric AD/HD.

Further investigations into therapies that do not have side effects or adverse reaction profiles like the current range of medications are recommended. Research of psychosocial, complementary and alternative interventions for the treatment and management of paediatric AD/HD would be the obvious choice. If research into CAM therapies can establish CAM as an evidence-based therapy for paediatric AD/HD then this may lead to an integrative approach where a combination of allopathic and alternative interventions may become the way forward. By utilising both paradigms this could potentially lead to decreasing dosages, frequency and duration of psychopharmaceuticals for children who have been prescribed AD/HD medications.

REFERENCES

[1] Wolraich M. Attention deficit hyperactivity disorder : the most studied and yet most controversial diagnosis. *Ment. Retard. Dev. Dis. Res. Rev.* 1999;5:163-168.

[2] American Psychiatric Association. *Diagnostic and Statistical Manual of Mental Disorders, Fourth Edition, Text Revision.* Washington DC: American Psychiatric Association; 2000.

[3] Barkley RA. *Attention-Deficit Hyperactivity Disorder:A Handbook for Diagnosis and Treatment.* Third ed. New York, NY: The Guilford Press; 2006.

[4]   Biederman J, Faraone SV. Attention-deficit hyperactivity disorder. *Lancet.* 2005;
        366(9481):237-248.

[5]   Rapport MD, Chung KM, Shore G, Denney CB, Isaacs P. Upgrading the science and
        technology of assessment and diagnosis: laboratory and clinic based assessment of
        children with ADHD. *J. Clin. Child Psychol.* 2000;29(4):555-569.

[6]   American Academy of Pediatrics. Clinical Practice Guideline: Diagnosis and
        Evaluation of the Child With Attention-Deficit/Hyperactivity Disorder. *Pediatrics.* May
        2000;105(5):1158-1170.

[7]   Brown RT, Freeman WS, Perrin JM, et al. Prevalence and Assessment of Attention-
        Deficit/Hyperactivity Disorder in Primary Care Settings. *Pediatrics.* 2001;107(3):E43.

[8]   Sawyer MG, Arney FM, Baghurst PA, et al. The mental health of young people in
        Australia: key findings from the child and adolescent component of the national survey
        of mental health and well being. *Aust. NZ. J. Psychiatry.* 2001;35(6):806-814.

[9]   Eiraldi RB, Power TJ, Karustis JL, Goldstein SG. Assessing ADHD and comorbid
        disorders in children: the Child Behavior Checklist and the Devereux Scales of Mental
        Disorders. *J. Clin. Child Psychol.* 2000;29(1):3-16.

[10]   Sørensen MJ, Mors O, Thomsen P. DSM-IV or ICD-10-DCR diagnoses in child and
        adolescent psychiatry: does it matter? *Eur. Child Adolesc. Psychiatry.* 2005;14(6):335-
        340.

[11]   Mezzich JE. International surveys on the use of ICD-10 and related diagnostic systems.
        Psychopathology. 2002;35(2-3):72-75.

[12]   Mayes R, Bagwell C, Erkulwater J. ADHD and the rise in stimulant use among
        children. *Harv. Rev. Psychiatry.* May-Jun 2008;16(3):151-166.

[13]   National Institute for Health and Clinical Excellence. *Attention Deficit Hyperactivity
        Disorder: The NICE Guideline on Diagnosis and Management of ADHD in Children,
        Young People and Adults.* Great Britain: The British Psychological Society and The
        Royal College of Psychiatrists; 2009.

[14]   National Institutes of Health. National Institutes of Health Consensus Development
        Conference Statement: Diagnosis and Treatment of Attention-Deficit/Hyperactivity
        Disorder (ADHD). *J. Am. Acad. Child Adolesc. Psychiatry.* 2000;39(2):182-193.

[15]   National Institutes of Health. NIH Consensus Statement : Diagnosis and treatment of
        attention deficit hyperactivity disorder (ADHD). 1998; http://www.ncbi.nlm.nih.gov/
        books/bv.fcgi?rid=hstat4.chapter.19663. Accessed 16th March 2009.

[16]   Wolraich ML, Wilson DB, White JW. The effect of sugar on behavior or cognition in
        children. A meta-analysis. *JAMA.* 1995;274(20):1617-1621.

[17]   Dulcan M, Dunne JE, Ayers W, et al. Practice parameters for the assessment and
        treatment of children, adolescents and adults with Attention Deficit/Hyperactivity
        Disorder. *J. Am. Acad. Child. Adolesc. Psychiatry.* 1997;36(10):85S-121S.

[18]   Johnston C, Leung D. Effects of medication, behavioral, and combined treatments on
        parents' and children's attributions for the behavior of children with attention-deficit
        hyperactivity disorder. *J. Consult. Clin. Psychol.* 2001;69(1):67-76.

[19]   DuPaul GJ. Assessment of ADHD symptoms:Comment on Gomez et al (2003).
        Psychol. Assess. 2003;15(1):115-117.

[20]   Naglieri J, Goldstein S, Delauder B, Schwebach A. Relationships between the WISC-III
        and the Cognitive Assessment System with Conners' Rating Scales and continuous
        performance tests. *Arch. Clin. Neuropsych.* 2005;20:385-401.

[21] Parens E, Johnston J. Facts, values, and Attention-Deficit Hyperactivity Disorder (ADHD): an update on the controversies. *Child Adol. Psychiatry Ment. Health.* 2009;3(1).

[22] Jadad AR, Booker L, Gauld M, et al. The treatment of attention-deficit hyperactivity disorder: an annotated bibliography and critical appraisal of published systematic reviews and meta-analyses. *Can. J. Psychiatry- Revue Canadienne de Psychiatrie.* 1999;44(10):1025-1035.

[23] Waslick B, Greenhill LL. Attention-Deficit/Hyperactivity Disorder. In: Wiener J, Dulcan M, eds. *Textbook of Child and Adolescent Psychiatry. 3rd edition.* Washington, DC: American Psychiatric Publishing; 2004:485-508.

[24] American Academy of Child and Adolescent Psychiatry. Practice Parameter for the Assessment and Treatment of Children and Adolescents with Attention-Deficit/Hyperactivity Disorder *J. Am. Acad. Child Adolesc. Psychiatry.* 2007; 46(7): 894-921.

[25] Brams M, Muniz R, Childress A, et al. A Randomized, Double-Blind, Crossover Study of Once-Daily Dexmethylphenidate in Children with Attention-Deficit Hyperactivity Disorder Rapid Onset of Effect. *CNS Drugs.* 2008;22(8):693-704.

[26] Schachter H, Pham B, King J, Langford S, Moher D. How efficacious and safe is short-acting methylphenidate for the treatment of attention-deficit disorder in children and adolescents? A meta-analysis. *Can. Med. Assoc. J.* 2001;165(11):1475-1488.

[27] Pelham WE, Wheeler T, Chronis A. Empirically supported psychosocial treatments for attention deficit hyperactivity disorder. *J. Clin. Child Psychol.* 1998;27(2):190-205.

[28] Chan E. The Role of Complementary and Alternative Medicine in Attention-Deficit Hyperactivity Disorder. *J. Dev. Behav. Pediatr.* 2002;23(1S):S37-S45.

[29] Arnold L. Treatment alternatives for attention-deficit/hyperactivity disorder (ADHD). *J. Atten. Disord.* 1999;3(1):30-48.

[30] Wilens TE, Adler LA, Adams J, et al. Misuse and Diversion of Stimulants Prescribed for ADHD: A Systematic Review of the Literature. *J. Am. Acad. Child Adolesc. Psychiatry.* 2008;47(1):21-31.

[31] Kutcher S, Aman M, Brooks SJ, et al. International consensus statement on attention-deficit/hyperactivity disorder (ADHD) and disruptive behaviour disorders (DBDs): clinical implications and treatment practice suggestions. *Eur. Neuropsychopharmacol.* 2004;14(1):11-28.

[32] Jensen P. Longer term effects of stimulant treatments for Attention-Deficit /Hyper-activity Disorder. *J. Atten. Disord.* 2002;6 Suppl 1:S45-56.

[33] Royal Australasian College of Physicians. Draft Systematic Review for the Guidelines on Attention Deficit Hyperactivity Disorder (ADHD) 2008; http://www.racp.edu.au/. Accessed 2009 Mar 16.

[34] American Academy of Pediatrics, and Subcommittee on Attention-Deficit/Hyper-activity Disorder and Committe on Quality Improvement. Clinical Practice Guideline: Treatment of the School Aged Child with Attention-Deficit/Hyperactivity Disorder. *Pediatrics.* 2001;108(4):1033-1044.

[35] Fabiano G, Pelham WE, Jr., Coles EK, Gnagy EM, Chronis-Tuscano A, O'Connor BC. A meta-analysis of behavioral treatments for attention-deficit/hyperactivity disorder. *Clin. Psychol. Rev.* 2009;29(2):129-140.

[36] Daughton JM, Kratochvil CJ. Review of ADHD pharmacotherapies: advantages, disadvantages, and clinical pearls. *J. Am. Acad. Child Adolesc. Psychiatry.* Mar 2009;48(3):240-248.

[37] Antshel K, Barkley R. Psychosocial Interventions in Attention Deficit Hyperactivity Disorder. *Child Adolesc. Psychiatr. Clin. N. Am.* 2008;17(2):421-437.

[38] Barbaresi WJ, Katusic SK, Colligan RC, Weaver AL, Leibson CL, Jacobsen SJ. Long-Term Stimulant Medication Treatment of Attention-Deficit/Hyperactivity Disorder: Results from a Population-Based Study. *J. Dev. Behav. Pediatr.* 2006;27(1):1-10.

[39] Chronis AM, Jones HA, Raggi VL. Evidence-based psychosocial treatments for children and adolescents with attention-deficit/hyperactivity disorder. *Clin. Psychol. Rev.* 2006;26(4):486-502.

[40] Brown RT, Amler RW, Freeman WS, et al. Treatment of Attention-Deficit/ Hyperactivity Disorder: Overview of the Evidence. *Pediatrics.* 2005;115(6):e749-e757.

[41] March JS, Swanson JM, Arnold LE, et al. Anxiety as a predictor and outcome variable in the multimodal treatment study of children with ADHD (MTA). *J. Abnorm. Child Psychol.* 2000;28(6):527-541.

[42] Conners CK. Forty years of methylphenidate treatment in Attention-Deficit/ Hyperactivity Disorder. *J. Atten. Disord.* 2002;6(Suppl 1):S17-30.

[43] Jensen PS, Hinshaw SP, Swanson JM, et al. Findings from the NIMH Multimodal Treatment Study of ADHD (MTA): implications and applications for primary care providers. *J. Dev. Behav. Pediatr.* Feb 2001;22(1):60-73.

[44] MTA Cooperative Group. A 14-Month Randomized Clinical Trial of Treatment Strategies for Attention-Deficit/ Hyperactivity Disorder. *Arch. Gen. Psychiatry.* 1999;56(12):1073-1086.

[45] Manos MJ, Tom-Revzon C, Bukstein OG, Crismon ML. Changes and challenges: managing ADHD in a fast-paced world. *J. Manage Care Pharm.* Nov 2007;13(9 Suppl B):S2-S13; quiz S14-S16.

[46] Kaiser NM, Hoza B, Hurt EA. Multimodal treatment for childhood attention-deficit/hyperactivity disorder. *Expert. Rev. Neurother.* 2008;8(10):1573-1583.

[47] Kendall T, Taylor E, Perez A, Taylor C, on behalf of the Guideline Development Group. Diagnosis and management of attention-deficit/hyperactivity disorder in children, young people, and adults: summary of NICE guidance. *Br. Med. J.* Sept 2008;337:a1239.

[48] Sonuga-Barke EJ. Categorical models of childhood disorder: a conceptual and empirical analysis. *J. Child Psychol. Psyc.* Jan 1998;39(1):115-133.

[49] Barbaresi WJ, Katusic SK, Colligan RC, Weaver AL, Jacobsen SJ. Long-Term School Outcomes for Children with Attention-Deficit/Hyperactivity Disorder: A Population-Based Perspective. *J. Dev. Behav. Pediatr.* 2007;28(4):265-273.

[50] Centers for Disease Control and Prevention. Mental health in the United States. Prevalence of diagnosis and medication treatment for attention-deficit/hyperactivity disorder--United States, 2003. *MMWR - Morbidity and Mortality Weekly Report.* Sep 2 2005;54(34):842-847.

[51] Olfson M, Gameroff MJ, Marcus SC, Jensen PS. National Trends in the Treatment of Attention Deficit Hyperactivity Disorder. *Am. J. Psychiatry.* Jun 2003;160(6):1071-1077.

[52] Rowland AS, Lesesne CA, Abramowitz AJ. The epidemiology of attention-deficit/ hyperactivity disorder (ADHD): a public health view. *Ment. Retard. Dev. Disabil. Res. Rev.* 2002;8(3):162-170.

[53] Barkley RA. *Attention Deficit Hyperactivity Disorder: A Handbook for Diagnosis and Treatment. 2nd ed.* New York: The Guilford Press; 1998a.

[54] Kollins SH, Shapiro SK, Newland MC, Abramowitz A. Discriminative and Participant-Rated Effects of Methylphenidate in Children Diagnosed With Attention Deficit Hyperactivity Disorder (ADHD). *Exp. Clin. Psychopharmacol.* 1998;6(4):375-389.

[55] Lerner M, Wigal T. Long-Term Safety of Stimulant Medications Used to Treat Children with ADHD. *Pediatr. Ann.* Jan 2008;37(1):37-45.

[56] Greenhill LL. The science of stimulant abuse. *Pediatr. Ann.* Aug 2006;35(8):552-556.

[57] Doggett MA. ADHD and Drug Therapy: is it Still a Valid Treatment? *J. Child Health Care.* 2004;8(1):69-81.

[58] Biederman J, Spencer T. Non-Stimulant treatments for ADHD. *Eur. Child Adolesc. Psychiatry.* 2000;9(Suppl 1):I51-I59.

[59] Van der Oord S, Prins PJM, Oosterlaan J, Emmelkamp PMG. Efficacy of methylphenidate, psychosocial treatments and their combination in school-aged children with ADHD: a meta-analysis. *Clin. Psychol. Rev.* Jun 2008;28(5):783-800.

[60] King S, Griffin S, Hodges Z, et al. A systematic review and economic model of the effectiveness and cost-effectiveness of methylphenidate, dexamfetamine and atomoxetine for the treatment of attention deficit hyperactivity disorder in children and adolescents. *Health Technol. Assess.* Jul 2006;10(23):iii-iv, xiii-146.

[61] Schachar R, Jadad AR, Gauld M, et al. Attention-Deficit Hyperactivity Disorder: Critical Appraisal of Extended Treatment Studies. *Can. J. Psychiatry- Revue Canadienne de Psychiatrie.* 2002;47(4):337-348.

[62] Klassen A, Miller A, Raina P, Lee SK, Olsen L. Attention-deficit hyperactivity disorder in children and youth: a quantitative systematic review of the efficacy of different management strategies. *Canadian Journal of Psychiatry - Revue Canadienne de Psychiatrie.* Dec 1999;44(10):1007-1016.

[63] Jensen PS, Arnold LE, Swanson JM, et al. 3-year follow-up of the NIMH MTA study. *J. Am. Acad. Child Adolesc. Psychiatry.* Aug 2007;46(8):989-1002.

[64] Poulton A. Growth and sexual maturation in children and adolescents with attention deficit hyperactivity disorder. *Curr. Opin. Pediatr.* 2006;18:427-434.

[65] dosReis S, Myers MA. Parental attitudes and involvement in psychopharmacological treatment for ADHD: a conceptual model. *Int. Rev. Psychiatry.* 2008;20(2):135-141.

[66] Pliszka SR. Non-stimulant treatment of attention-deficit/hyperactivity disorder. *CNS Spectr.* Apr 2003;8(4):253-258.

[67] Rapport MD, Moffitt C. Attention deficit/hyperactivity disorder and methylphenidate. A review of height/weight, cardiovascular, and somatic complaint side effects. *Clin. Psychol. Rev.* 2002;22(8):1107-1131.

[68] Ministerial Implementation Committee for Attention Deficit Hyperactivity Disorder in Western Australia (MICADHD), Telethon Institute for Child Health Research (TICHR). Raine ADHD Study: Long-term outcomes associated with stimulant medication in the treatment of ADHD in children In: Department of Health, ed: Government of Western Australia; 2010.

[69] Pelham WE, Jr, , Gnagy EM. Psychosocial and combined treatments for ADHD. *Ment. Retard. Dev. Disabil. Res. Rev.* 1999a;5(3):225-236.

[70] Miranda A, Jarque S, Rosel J. Treatment of children with ADHD: Psychopedagogical program at school verses psychostimulant medication. *Psichothema.* 2006;18(3):335-341.

[71] Bukstein OG. Satisfaction with Treatment for Attention-Deficit/Hyperactivity Disorder. *Am. J. Manag. Care.* Jul 2004;10(4 Suppl):S107-116.

[72] Root RW, Resnick RJ. An update on the diagnosis and treatment of attention-deficit/hyperactivity disorder in children. *Prof. Psychol: Res. Pr.* 2003;34(1):34-41.

[73] Sinha D, Efron D. Complementary and alternative medicine use in children with attention deficit hyperactivity disorder. *J. Paediatr. Child Health.* Jan-Feb 2005 2005;41:(1-2):23-26.

[74] Eisenberg DM, Davis RB, Ettner SL, et al. Trends in alternative medicine use in the United States, 1990-97: Results of a follow up survey. *JAMA.* 1998;280(18):1569-1575.

[75] Rojas N, Chan E. Old and new controversies in the alternative treatment of attention-deficit hyperactivity disorder. *Ment. Retard. Dev. Dis. Res. Rev.* 2005;11(2):116-130.

[76] Sawni-Sikand A, Schubiner H, Thomas RL. Use of complementary/alternative therapies among children in primary care pediatrics. *Ambul. Pediatr.* Mar-Apr 2002;2(2):99-103.

[77] Kemper K, Vohra S, Walls R. The use of complementary and alternative medicine in pediatrics. *Pediatrics.* Dec 2008;122(6):1374-1386.

[78] Spigelblatt L, Laine-Ammara G, Pless IB, Guyver A. The use of alternative medicine by children. *Pediatrics.* Dec 1994;94(6 Pt 1):811-814.

[79] National Health Service (NHS) Evidence. Complementary and Alternative Medicine. 2008; http://www.library.nhs.uk/cam/Page.aspx? pagename=LIBDEV. Accessed 17th Sept, 2009.

[80] Manheimer E, Berman B. Cochrane Complementary Medicine Field. *About The Cochrane Collaboration* (Fields) 2009(Issue 2. Art. No.: CE000052).

[81] South M, Lim A. Use of complementary and alternative medicine in children:Too important to ignore. *J. Paediatr. Child Health.* 2003;39(8):573-574.

[82] Baumgaertel A. Alternative and controversial treatments for attention-deficit/hyperactivity disorder. *Pediatr. Clin. North. Am.* 1999;46(5):977-992.

[83] Brue AW, Oakland TD. Alternative treatments for attention-deficit/hyperactivity disorder: does evidence support their use? *Altern. Ther. Health Med.* 2002;8(1):68-70.

[84] Chan E, Rappaport L, Kemper K. Complementary and alternative therapies in childhood attention and hyperactivity problems. *J. Dev. Behav. Pediatr.* Feb 2003;24(1):4-8.

[85] Sawni A. Attention-deficit/hyperactivity disorder and complementary/ alternative medicine. *Adolesc. Med.* 2008;19(2):313-326.

[86] Bush G, Valera EM, Seidman LJ. Functional neuroimaging of attention-deficit/ hyper activity disorder: A review and suggested future directions. *Biol. Psychiatry.* 2005;57(11):1273-1284.

[87] Gross-Tsur V, Lahad A, Shalev R. Use of Complementary Medicine in Children With Attention Deficit Hyperactivity Disorder and Epilepsy. *Pediatr. Neurol.* July 2003;29(1):53-55.

[88] Stubberfield T, Wray J, Parry T. Utilization of alternative therapies in attention-deficit hyperactivity disorder. *J. Pediatr. Child Health.* 1999;35:450-453.

[89] Bussing R, Zima BT, Gary FA, Garvan CW. Use of Complementary and Alternative Medicine for Symptoms of Attention-Deficit Hyperactivity Disorder. *Psychiatr. Serv.* 2002;53(9):1096-1102.

[90] National Centre for Complementary and Alternative Medicine. *CAM use and Children.* 2007; http://nccam.nih.gov/health/children/. Accessed 17th Sept, 2009.

[91] Barnes PM, Bloom B, Nahin RL. Complementary and alternative medicine use among adults and children: United States, 2007. *Natl. Health Stat. Report.* Dec 10 2008(12):1-23.

[92] Daley KC. Update on attention-deficit/hyperactivity disorder. *Curr. Opin. Pediatr.* Apr 2004;16(2):217-226.

[93] Yussman SM, Ryan SA, Auinger P, Weitzman M. Visits to complementary and alternative medicine providers by children and adolescents in the United States. *Ambul. Pediatr.* Sep-Oct 2004;4(5):429-435.

[94] Richardson A, Montgomery P. The Oxford-Durham study: a randomized, controlled trial of dietary supplementation with fatty acids in children with developmental coordination disorder. *Pediatrics.* 2005;115(5):1360-1366.

[95] Sinn N, Bryan J. Effect of supplementation with polyunsaturated fatty acids and micronutrients on ADHD-related problems with attention and behavior. *J. Dev. Behav. Pediatr.* Jan 2007a;28(2):82-91.

[96] Richardson AJ. Omega-3 fatty acids in ADHD and related neurodevelopmental disorders. *Int. Rev. Psychiatry.* 2006;18(2):155-172.

[97] Richardson AJ, Ross MA. Fatty acid metabolism in neurodevelopmental disorder: a new perspective on associations between attention-deficit/hyperactivity disorder, dyslexia, dyspraxia and the autistic spectrum. *Prostaglandins Leukotr. Essent. Fatty Acids.* 2000a;63(1-2):1-9.

[98] Hallahan B, Garland MR. Essential fatty acids and their role in the treatment of impulsivity disorders. *Prostaglandins Leukot. Essent. Fatty Acids.* 2004;71:211-216.

[99] Stevens L, Zhang W, Peck L, et al. EFA supplementation in children with inattention, hyperactivity, and other disruptive behaviors. *Lipids.* 2003;38(10):1007-1021.

[100] Richardson AJ. Clinical trials of fatty acid treatment in ADHD, dyslexia, dyspraxia and the autistic spectrum. *Prostaglandins Leukotrienes and Essential Fatty Acids.* Apr 2004a;70(4):383-390.

[101] Richardson AJ, Puri BK. A randomized double-blind, placebo-controlled study of the effects of supplementation with highly unsaturated fatty acids on ADHD-related symptoms in children with specific learning difficulties. *Prog. Neuropsychopharmacol. Biol. Psychiatry.* Feb 2002;26(2):233-239.

[102] Hirayama S, Hamazaki T, Terasawa K. Effect of docosahexaenoic acid-containing food administration on symptoms of attention-deficit/hyperactivity disorder - a placebo-controlled double-blind study. *Eur. J. Clin. Nutr.* 2004;58(3):467-473.

[103] Voigt R, Llorente A, Jensen C, Fraley J, Berretta M, Heird W. A randomized, double-blind, placebo-controlled trial of docosahexaenoic acid supplementation in children with attention-deficit/hyperactivity disorder. *J. Paediatr.* 2001;139(2):189-196.

[104] Arnold LE, Pinkham SM, Votolato NA. Does zinc moderate essential fatty acid and amphetamine treatment of attention-deficit/ hyperactivity disorder? *J. Child Adolesc. Psychopharmacol.* 2000;10:111-117.

[105] Richardson AJ. Long-chain polyunsaturated fatty acids in childhood developmental and psychiatric disorders. *Lipids.* Dec 2004b;39(12):1215-1222.

[106] Richardson AJ, Puri BK. The potential role of fatty acids in attention-deficit/hyper-activity disorder. *Prostaglandins Leukotrienes and Essential Fatty Acids.* Jul-Aug 2000b;63(1-2):79-87.

[107] Raz R, Gabis L. Essential fatty acids and attention-deficit-hyperactivity disorder: a systematic review. *Dev. Med. Child Neurol.* Aug 2009;51(8):580-592.

[108] Furman L. What Is Attention-Deficit Hyperactivity Disorder (ADHD)? *J. Child Neurol.* 2005;20(12):994-1002.

[109] Kaplan BJ, Dewey DM, Crawford SG, Wilson BN. The term comorbidity is of questionable value in reference to developmental disorders: data and theory. *J. Learn Disabil.* 2001;34(6):555-565.

[110] Arnold LE. Alternative treatments for adults with attention-deficit hyperactivity disorder (ADHD). *Ann. N. Y. Acad. Sci.* Jun Jun 2001;931:310-341.

[111] Feingold BE. *Why Your Child is Hyperactive.* New York: Random House; 1975.

[112] Kavale K, Forness SR. Hyperactivity and Diet Treatment: A Meta-Analysis of the Feingold Hypothesis *J. Learn Disabil.* 1983;16(6):324-330.

[113] Williams JI, Cram DM. Diet in the management of hyperkinesis: A review of the tests of Feingold's hypotheses. *Can. Psychiatr. Assoc. J.* 1978;23:241-248.

[114] Mattes JA. The Feingold diet: A current reappraisal. *J. Learn Disabil.* 1983;16:319-323.

[115] Wender EH. The food additive–free diet in the treatment of behavior disorders: A review. *J. Behav. Pediatr.* 1986;7:35-42.

[116] Howard AL, Robinson M, Smith GJ, Ambrosini GL, Piek JP, Oddy WH. ADHD Is Associated With a 'Western' Dietary Pattern in Adolescents. *J. Atten. Disord.* 2011;15(5):403-411.

[117] Ambrosini GL, Oddy WH, Robinson M, et al. Adolescent dietary patterns are associated with lifestyle and family psychosocial factors. *Public Health Nutrition.* 2009;12(10).

[118] Monastra VJ, Lynn S, Linden M, Lubar JF, Gruzelier J, LaVaque TJ. Electro-encephalographic biofeedback in the treatment of attention-deficit/hyperactivity disorder. *Appl. Psychophysiol. Biofeedback.* Jun 2005 2005;30(2):95-114.

[119] Thompson L, Thompson M. Neurofeedback combined with training in metacognitive strategies: effectiveness in students with ADD. *Appl. Psychophysiol. Biofeedback.* 1998;23(4):243-263.

[120] Frei H, Everts R, von Ammon K, et al. Homeopathic treatment of children with attention deficit hyperactivity disorder: a randomised, double blind, placebo controlled crossover trial. *Eur. J. Pediatr.* Jul 2005 2005;164(12):758-767.

[121] Heirs M, Dean ME. Homeopathy for attention deficit/hyperactivity disorder or hyperkinetic disorder. *Cochrane Database of Syst Rev.* 2007(4):Art. No.: CD005648. DOI: 005610.001002/14651858. CD14005648.pub14651852.

[122] Coulter MK, Dean ME. Homeopathy for attention deficit/hyperactivity disorder or hyperkinetic disorder. *Cochrane Database of Syst. Rev.* 2007(4):CD005648.

[123] Lamont J. Homeopathic treatment of attention deficit disorder *Br. Homeopath J.* 1997;86:196-200.

[124] Strauss L. The efficacy of a homeopathic preparation in the management of attention deficit hyperactivity disorder. *Biol. Ther.* 2000;18:197-201.

[125] Jacobs J, Williams A-L, Girard C, Njike VY, Katz D. Homeopathy for attention-deficit/hyperactivity disorder: a pilot randomized-controlled trial.[see comment]. *J. Altern. Complement Med.* Oct 2005;11(5):799-806.

[126] Barkley RA. Attention Deficit Hyperactivity Disorder: *A Handbook for Diagnosis and Treatment.* New York: The Guilford Press; 1990.

[127] Field T, Quintino O, Hernandez-Reif M. Adolescents with attention deficit hyperactivity disorder benefit from massage therapy. *Adolescence.* 1998;33:103-108.

[128] Field T. Massage Therapy Effects. *Am. Psychol.* 1998;53(12):1270-1281.

[129] Maddigan B, Hodgson P, Heath S, et al. The effects of massage therapy and exercise therapy on children/adolescents with attention deficit hyperactivity disorder. *Can. Child Adol. Psychaitry Rev.* Mar 2003;12(2):40-43.

[130] World Health Organization. *World Health Organization (WHO) guidelines on basic training and safety in chiropractic.* 2005; http://apps.who.int/medicinedocs /en/m/ abstract/Js14076e/. Accessed 2009 Mar 16.

[131] World Federation of Chiropractic (WFC). http://www.wfc.org/ website/WFC/ website.nsf/. Accessed December 10, 2009.

[132] Bergmann TF. Chiropractic Technique. In: Gatterman MI, ed. *Foundations of Chiropractic*:Subluxation Second Edition. Vol Second Edition. Philadelphia, PA: Mosby Inc.; 2005.

[133] Palmer D. *The science, art, and philosophy of chiropractic.* Portlan, OR: Portland Printing House; 1910.

[134] Pitetti R, Singh S, Hornyak D, Garcia SE, Herr S. Complementary and alternative medicine use in children. *Pediatr. Emerg. Care.* Jun 2001;17(3):165-169.

[135] Wolsko PM, Eisenberg DM, Davis RB, Kessler R, Phillips RS. *Patterns and perceptions of care for treatment of back and neck pain: results of a national survey.* Spine. Feb 1 2003;28(3):292-297; discussion 298.

[136] Alcantara J. The presenting complaints of pediatric patients for chiropractic care: Results from a practice-based research network. *Clin. Chiropr.* 2008;11:193-198.

[137] Jamison J, Davies N. Paediatric Patients Seeking Chiropractic Care: An Australian Case Study. *Chiropr. J.* Aust. 2005;35:143-146.

[138] Walker S, Bablis P, Pollard H, McHardy A. Practitioner Perceptions of Emotions Associated with Pain: *A Survey. J. Chiropr. Med.* 2005;4(1):11-18.

[139] Walker S. *Neuro Emotional Technique: N.E.T. Basic Seminar Manual.* Encinatas, CA, USA: N.E.T Inc; 1996.

[140] Bablis P, Pollard H, Bonello R. A retrospective analysis of self-reported symptoms from 761 consecutive new patients presenting to a Neuro Emotional Technique chiropractic clinic. *Complement Ther. Clin. Pract.* 2009;15(3):166-171.

[141] Hawk C, Khorsan R, Lisi AJ, Ferrance RJ, Evans MW. Chiropractic care for nonmusculoskeletal conditions: a systematic review with implications for whole systems research. *J. Altern. Complement Med.* 2007;13(5):491-512.

[142] Karpouzis F, Bonello R, Pollard H. Chiropractic care for paediatric and adolescent Attention-Deficit/Hyperactivity Disorder: A systematic review. Chiropr Osteopat. 2010;18:13.

[143] Wittman R, Vallone S, Williams K. Chiropractic management of six-year-old child with attention deficit hyperactivity disorder (ADHD). J Clin Chiropr Pediatr. 2009;10(1):612-20.

[144] Cassista G. Improvement in a child with Attention Deficit Hyperactivity Disorder, Kyphotic Cervical Curve and Vertebral Subluxation Undergoing Chiropractic Care. J Vert Sublux Res. 2009(April 20):1-5.

[145] Bedell L. Successful care of a young female with ADD/ADHD and vertebral subluxation: a case study. J Vert Sublux Res. 2008(June 23):1-7.

[146] Young A. Chiropractic management of a child with ADD/ADHD. J Vert Sublux Res. 2007(Sept 6):1-4.

[147] Lovett L, Blum C. Behavioral and Learning Changes Secondary to Chiropractic Care to Reduce Subluxations in a Child with Attention Deficit Hyperactivity Disorder: A Case Study. J Vert Sublux Res. 2006(Oct 4):1-6.

[148] Bastecki A, Harrison D, Haas JW. Cervical Kyphosis Is a Possible Link to Attention-Deficit/Hyperactivity Disorder. J Manipulative Physiol Ther. 2004;27(8):525e1-e5.

[149] Elster EL. Upper cervical chiropractic care for a nine-year-old male with Tourette syndrome, attention deficit hyperactivity disorder, depression, asthma, insomnia, and headaches: a case report. J Vert Sublux Res. 2003 Jul 12;12:1-11.

[150] Stone-McCoy PA, Przybysz L. Chiropractic Management of a Child with Attention Deficit Hyperactivity Disorder & Vertebral Subluxation: A Case Study. J Pediatr Maternal & Family Health - Chiropr. 2009(1):1-8.

[151] Liesman NJ. A Case Study of ADHD. ICA Review. 1998 Oct;54:54-61.

[152] Peet J. Adjusting the hyperactive/ADD pediatric patient. Chiropr Pediatr. 1997;2(4):12-6.

[153] Peet P. Child with chronic illness: Respiratory infections, ADHD, and fatigue response to Chiropractic Care. Chiropr Pediatr. 1997;3(1):12-3.

[154] Barnes T. A multi-faceted chiropractic approach to attention deficit hyperactivity disorder: a case report. Int Chiropr Assoc. 1995 Jan/Feb:41-3.

[155] Barnes T. Not a Cookie Cutter Problem: Attention Deficit Hyperactivity Disorder. Dynamic Chiropr. 1994;12(11):1-7.

[156] Langley C. Epileptic seizures, Nocturnal enuresis and Attention Deficit Disorder. Chiropr Pediatr. 1994;1(1).

[157] Andersen C, Partridge J. Seizures plus Attention Deficit Hyperactivity Disorder: A case report. Int Chiropr Assoc. 1993;49(4):35-7.

[158] Pauli Y. Improvement in attention in patients undergoing network spinal analysis: A case series using objective measures of attention. J Vert Sublux Res. 2007b(Aug 23):1-9.

[159] Pauli Y. ADHD research project collects case study reports. Chiropr J. 2007a Jan 2007;21(4):1, 36.

[160] Mileski M, McClay R. The Role of Chiropractic in the Treatment of ADHD. Dynamic Chiropr. 2003;21(5):1-6.

[161] Giesen JM, Center DB, Leach RA. An evaluation of chiropractic manipulation as a treatment of hyperactivity in children. J Manipulative Physiol Ther. 1989;12(5):353-63.

[162] Goff P, Sheader WE, Sheader DF, Thornton M. Using a computerized continuous performance test to assess the effects of chiropractic adjustment on attention span: A pilot study. Chiropr J Aust. 2000;30(2):48-54.

[163] Brzozowske W, Walton E. The effect of chiropractic treatment on students with learning and behavioral impairments resulting form neurological dysfunction. J Aust Chiro Assoc. 1980;11(7):13-8.

[164] Brzozowske W, Walton E. The effect of chiropractic treatment on students with learning and behavioral impairments resulting form neurological dysfunction. J Aust Chiro Assoc. 1977;11(7):S127-S40.

[165] Karpouzis F, Bonello R, Pollard H. Final data of the effects of the Neuro Emotional Technique (NET) for pediatric Attention-Deficit/Hyperactivity Disorder (AD/HD): A randomized controlled trial. Clin Chiropr. 2011;14(4):144.

[166] Karpouzis F, Pollard H, Bonello R. A randomised controlled trial of the Neuro Emotional Technique (NET) for childhood Attention Deficit Hyperactivity Disorder (ADHD): a protocol. Trials. 2009;10(6).

[167] Maizes V, Rakel D, Niemiec C. Integrative medicine and patient-centered care. Explore (NY). 2009 Sep-Oct;5(5):277-89.

[168] Shannon S. Integrative approaches to pediatric mood disorders. Altern Ther Health Med. 2009 Sep-Oct;15(5):48-53.

[169] Kidd P. Attention Deficit/Hyperactivity Disorder (ADHD) in Children: Rationale for its Integrative Management. Altern Med Rev. 2000 Oct;5(5):402-28.

[170] Harding KL, Judah RD, Gant CE. Outcome-Based Comparison of Ritalin® versus Food-Supplement Treated Children with AD/HD. Altern Med Rev. 2003;8(3):319-30.

[171] Moher D, Soeken K, Sampson M, Ben-Porat L, Berman B. Assessing the quality of reports of randomized trials in pediatric complementary and alternative medicine. BMC Pediatrics. 2002;2(3):1-8.

[172] Sampson M, Campbell K, Ajiferuke I, Moher D. Randomized controlled trials in pediatric complementary and alternative medicine: where can they be found? BMC Pediatrics. 2003;3:1.

[173] Kemper KJ, O'Connor KG. Pediatricians' recommendations for complementary and alternative medical (CAM) therapies. Ambul Pediatr. 2004 Nov-Dec;4(6):482-7.

[174] Lawson ML, Pham B, Klassen TP, Moher D. Systematic reviews involving complementary and alternative medicine interventions had higher quality of reporting than conventional medicine reviews. J Clin Epidemiol. 2005 Aug;58(8):777-84.

In: Alternative Medicine
Editors: Kenneth R. Carter and George E. Murphy

ISBN 978-1-62257-106-2
©2012 Nova Science Publishers, Inc.

Chapter 4

CHRONICALLY ILL PATIENTS' EXPERIENCE OF ILLNESS AND HEALING RELATIONSHIPS IN INTEGRATIVE MEDICINE

Nathalie Richard
RBC – Life Sciences & Health Services
Samia Chreim
University of Ottawa, Canada
Ivy Lynn Bourgeault
University of Ottawa, Canada
Douglas E. Angus
University of Ottawa, Canada

ABSTRACT

The increasing incidence of chronic illness and the popularity of integrative medicine approaches as treatment modalities require that we better understand the meaning that chronically ill patients attribute to their illness and treatment experience. This paper is based on a phenomenological study that sought to understand how nine chronically ill patients perceived their experience of living with their illnesses and receiving treatment at an integrative medicine clinic situated in an urban centre in Canada. Participants' accounts of how they experienced their health and illness were framed as contrasts between their past and present selves. Their experience of their relationships with and care received from providers at the integrative clinic was framed against the backdrop of their experiences in conventional medicine contexts. The findings indicate that participants' illnesses disrupted their life and sense of self. Declining health and influence of members in their social milieu were impetuses for joining the clinic, where participants developed enriched relationships with clinicians. These relationships allowed them to feel cared for and empowered. Following treatments at the clinic, participants experienced improvements in their health status, a return to their old or renewed sense of self, and hope for the future. We provide rich data from the participants' interviews, and we consider the implications of living with and receiving treatment for chronic illness.

INTRODUCTION

Increasing longevity rates due to health care advances and an aging population have resulted in an increased number of individuals suffering from chronic illnesses. There has been sustained interest in how patients who suffer from chronic illness experience their conditions (Charmaz, 1983, 1995; Clare 2003; Ironside et al, 2003; Raheim & Haland, 2006). This stems from an increased awareness that patients often have unique perspectives on their illness that are not captured by more objectified descriptions. There has been a parallel increase in attention to patients' seeking of complementary and alternative medicine (CAM) and of integrative medicine (a combination of alternative and conventional treatments) to manage their chronic condition (Hok et al., 2007; Ohlen et al., 2006). CAM and integrative medicine's emphasis on wellness and holistic approaches represents an attractive treatment modality for patients seeking complex care (Bell et al., 2002). Given the growing use of complementary and integrative medicine, it is important that we understand the experiences of individuals who choose these treatment modalities. In this paper, we report on a phenomenological study of nine chronically ill patients' experiences of living with their illnesses and receiving treatment at an integrative medicine clinic.

Chronic illnesses often result not only in pain and emotional distress, but also poorer quality of life and changes in self-identity (Whittemore & Dixon, 2008). Chronic conditions alter the personal life story of the people that they affect. It is what Öhman et al. (2003) call a "break with the past" and a revision of future life goals. In his study of the chronically ill, Bury (1982) described this as a "biographical disruption" where participants had to reconstruct their life story and modify how they perceived their self. Chronic illness creates a sense of disorder in the life world and renders the individual vulnerable. The impairments that arise of these conditions require significant adjustments in daily living. As Charmaz (1983) pointed out, the physical and emotional consequences of the illness, and the demands of the treatments can negatively influence social activities. Social withdrawal, depression and feelings of becoming a burden can threaten the self. The self, as Baumesiter indicated, "encompasses the direct feeling each person has of privileged access to his or her own thoughts and feelings and sensations. It begins with the awareness of one's own body and is augmented by the sense of being able to make choices and initiate action" (1997:681). Given that chronic illness is experienced in the body and might be accompanied by debilitating effects which diminish the patient's ability to make choices, it can be understood why chronic illness can be experienced as a threat to the self.

Consistently with the increased focus on the self and the importance of giving patients a stronger voice in the management and control of their illness, self-management procedures have been garnering interest. Studies of the impact of illness representation on self-management procedures (e.g. Horowitz et al. 2004) reveal that patients often fail to recognize the chronic nature of their illness due to a lack of information on symptoms and causes of their illness, and that they do not have the tools necessary to manage their condition. Self-management programs can result in improvements in self-efficacy and quality of life (Smith et al., 2007).

An important component in how the self and self-management procedures are experienced is the relationship that the patient holds with the care provider. The physician-patient relationship, for example, has been well studied as central to those living with a chronic illness (Bury, 1982; Charmaz, 1983; Ohman et al., 2003). When information provided to patients by their physicians does not correspond with their own perception of their condition, this causes confusion; patients feel relief when the explanations are consistent with their perceptions (Öhman et al., 2003). In general, patients want to be seen more as individuals than a disease entity and as experts on their life (Haugli et al., 2004). Accepting patients' perspective is seen as contributing to a supportive physician-patient relationship.

Terms such as "collaborative care" (Wasson et al., 2006), "working alliances" (Fuertes et al., 2007), and "partnerships" (Goldring et al., 2002) point to the type of physician-patient relationship that is emerging as important. These terms refer to the inclusion of patients as active agents, able to exert control over their health. Collectively the above and other studies (e.g. Parchman et al., 2005; Kaplan et al., 1989) in the field of conventional medicine have pointed to the influence of physician-patient relationship and communication on patients' ability to achieve better health outcomes. Recent research in the context of integrative medicine has shown similar findings (Koithan et al., 2007). The elements that patients identify as crucial for a good physician-patient relationship are: listening and taking into consideration patient and family concerns, showing respect, spending enough time with patients, taking into consideration bio-psycho-social variables, treating the patient as a partner, and empowering the patient.

In sum, chronic illness has a major impact on the lives of patients and their sense of self. An important element of any treatment modality is the clinician-patient relationship since it can enable patients to exert control over their health condition and to live a more satisfying life. Patients may seek alternative or integrative medicine as a way to deal with their illness and to secure a more collaborative relationship with their provider. Given this, we attempted to understand the lived experience of chronically ill patients by asking how patients experience their illness and health before and after seeking treatments at an integrative clinic and how they experience their relationship with and the care they receive at the clinic.

METHODOLOGY

The study was inspired by interpretative phenomenology. Interpretative Phenomeno-logical Analysis (IPA) is concerned with understanding the meaning of individual experiences or phenomena from the perspective of the participants (J.A. Smith et al., 2009). The focus is on individuals' sense making of an experience within a specific context. Phenomenological researchers seek to uncover the meaning that individual participants attribute to their experience and then move from the particular (idiographic) to an analysis of the similarities and differences across participants in search for patterns in the experiences (Creswell, 2007; J.A. Smith et al., 2009). Due to the idiographic nature of IPA, it "utilizes small, purposively-selected and carefully-situated samples" (J.A. Smith et al., 2009:29); thus, there is a "narrow range of sampling strategies for a phenomenological study" (Creswell, 1997:128). Unlike nomothetic approaches, and similar to case studies, phenomenological analysis demonstrates existence and not frequency (J.A. Smith et al., 2009: Stake, 1995; Yin, 2009).

Research Setting

The study took place at an integrative clinic in an urban centre in Canada owned by a physician, whom we will call Dr. Smith, and who practices integrative medicine. In addition to the integrative physician, the clinic is operated by a team of five internationally-trained physicians (MD) who are completing training in order to receive a licence to practice in Canada. The clinic offers a combination of conventional and alternative medicine, as well as chelation therapy, which is used to supplement conventional treatments for patients with coronary heart disease or diabetes. The integration of the two treatment modalities occurs at the level of the physician-owner who is certified to deliver both conventional and alternative medicine. The integrative physician completed training for a medical degree as well as acupuncture and Chinese medicine. He is the author of several studies on alternative and integrative medicine and is a lecturer in the faculty of medicine at a Canadian university.

Data Collection

Access to participants was obtained by a member of the research team through the physician-owner. The participants were purposefully sampled— all were chronically ill patients and were receiving treatments at the integrative clinic. Patients interested in participating had to meet the following inclusion criteria: a) they had been patients at the clinic, b) they received alternative medical treatments on a regular basis, and c) they were between the ages of 18-80.

A recruitment letter was posted at the front desk of the clinic. The letter indicated that the researcher was seeking patients to participate in a study. Patients that responded to the letter and that met the eligibility criteria were selected on a first-come basis and gender did not factor into the selection process. The nine participants selected for the study consisted of eight men and one woman. Patients were assured that their participation would not impact delivery of care and that the results of the interview would be kept confidential. The patients who agreed to participate were assigned pseudonyms. Table 1 provides information on the participants. Interviews took place at the integrative clinic between April and August, 2009. One of the research team members conducted all the interviews, which lasted between 30 minutes and an hour. The interview was concluded when participants felt they had no further information to contribute. Participants were interviewed in a quiet, private area at a time that was convenient to them. An interview guide was used to help patients recount how they experienced their health and illness and the relationship with the clinic staff. The guide covered the following topics: a) how patients experienced their health condition prior to seeking treatment at the integrative clinic, b) what factors led patients to attend the clinic, c) how they experienced treatments and relationships with the staff at the clinic, and d) how they viewed the outcome of their treatment. Although a general interview guide was used, participants were free to describe the important elements of their experience, and the interviewer probed participants about their answers. All interviews were audio-recorded and transcribed verbatim. The study protocol received approval from the University's Research Ethics Board.

Table 1. Description of Participants

Patient	Age	Chronic illness	Length of time at the clinic	Frequency of time at the clinic
Cynthia	49	Type II diabetes, hypothyroidism	More than a year	Once a month
Marc	59	Angina, partially functioning heart following a heart attack	4 months	Once a week
Allan	77	Type II diabetes, heart palpitations	5 months	Once a week
David	65	Type II diabetes, hypothyroidism	3-4 years	Once a month
Daniel	62	Clogged arteries, high iron levels, type II diabetes and parasitic flu	3-4 weeks	Twice a week
Andre	70	Hypertension, shoulder pain	1 month	Once a week
Michael	60	Hypertension, previous heart attack	2 years	Twice a week
Robert	70	Hypertension, high levels of heavy metals	3 months	Once a month
Adam	67	Type II diabetes, hypertension	5 months	Twice a week

Data Analysis and Validation

Data collected from the interviews was analyzed using procedures outlined in interpretative phenomenological analysis (J.A. Smith et al., 2009) and qualitative research (Miles and Huberman, 1994). Analysis involved a careful reading of each of the transcripts, identification of meaning units, and writing descriptive and interpretive summaries of the participant's experiences (Miles and Huberman, 1994). Finding patterns between themes involved constructing files with transcript extracts for each theme, combining like with like in order to develop a more abstract name, or a pattern code for the cluster (Miles and Huberman, 1994; J.A. Smith et al., 2009). This process involved continued analysis of the data and discussion between two researchers in this study until agreement was achieved on the categories. (The categories are illustrated in Figure 1).

Assessing the validity and quality of the research includes evaluating sensitivity to context and rigour (J.A. Smith et al., 2009). These can be demonstrated in the researchers' empathy and engagement with the particular; the use of verbatim extracts that give participants a voice and allow readers to check the researchers' interpretations; an awareness of extant literature on methods and on the topic; choice of a research sample that matches the research questions; and commitment to the analysis apparent in moving beyond simple descriptions about individual participants to say something about the meanings of the themes they share. These elements were demonstrated in this study. Attention to context is shown through the collection and reporting of particular information on participants. Extensive quotes from participants are provided throughout the Findings section. Engagement with the extant literature is demonstrated in various sections of this paper. The results and the model reported attest to the particular in participants' experiences, but also move beyond the specific to emphasize patterns across experiences. Having different researchers working with the data set and agreeing on categories that were well grounded in the data is further indication of rigour (Miles and Huberan, 1994; Creswell, 2007).

FINDINGS

Figure 1 outlines the similarities in the experience of the participants. Participants described their experience of living with a chronic condition – prior to joining the integrative clinic – in negative terms. A disparity between their desired and current health status, combined with the influence of members in their social sphere instigated participants to join the clinic. At the clinic, they experienced being cared for and achieving empowerment due to the relationships they held with the clinic staff. Participants described positive experiences following the treatments at the clinic, which included a return to a more valued sense of self, expressed in better physical condition, and a much improved emotional, mental and social life.

Participants' Experience of their Chronic Condition Prior to Seeking Integrative *Care*

Experiences of chronic illness before seeking treatment at the integrative clinic included deterioration of physical appearance and energy level, inability to fulfill social responsibilities, and diminished social interactions. In a few cases, death wishes were expressed. Patients suffering from more severe forms of chronic illness expressed greater concern for their health and were more aware of the impact of the condition on their physical appearance and activities. Adam, for example, repeatedly referred to change in his physical appearance as represented by the loss of hair on his legs and by his hair turning white.

> Because I went to the point my hormones were low, I lost the hair from my leg. I didn't have... hair on my leg... I was white, my hair went really, really white.

Participants also spoke about experiencing restrictions in their daily activities and a decrease in their quality of life. The inability to complete routine activities such as regular work tasks, performing household chores, or driving, was a common theme. Restrictions in daily activities often reflected the lack of control that patients had over their condition.

For Cynthia, the illness affected her physical abilities:

> I used to have a lot of problems with my feet where I couldn't walk, where I was in a lot of pain.

The illness also challenged the image that some participants had of themselves within the family context. There were concerns about the inability to meet family responsibilities and the need to limit engagement. Daniel explained:

Experience of living with a chronic condition: diminished self
-Negative change in physical appearance
-Reduced physical energy level
-Social withdrawal
-Death imagery

Impetus
-Lack of improvement or deterioration of health status
-Social influence

Experiences at the integrative clinic

Feeling cared for
-Empathy and availability of staff
-Thoroughness of service provision

Feeling empowered
-Being informed
-Achieving control over health
-Ability to make decisions
-Achieving health objectives

Contrasting images of conventional and integrative medicine

Relationships with integrative physician and clinic staff

Contrasting images of past and present

Impact: return to a former, more valued self
-Positive change in physical appearance
-Improved physical energy level
-Emotional, mental and social wellbeing
-Hope
-Setting and achieving life/future goals

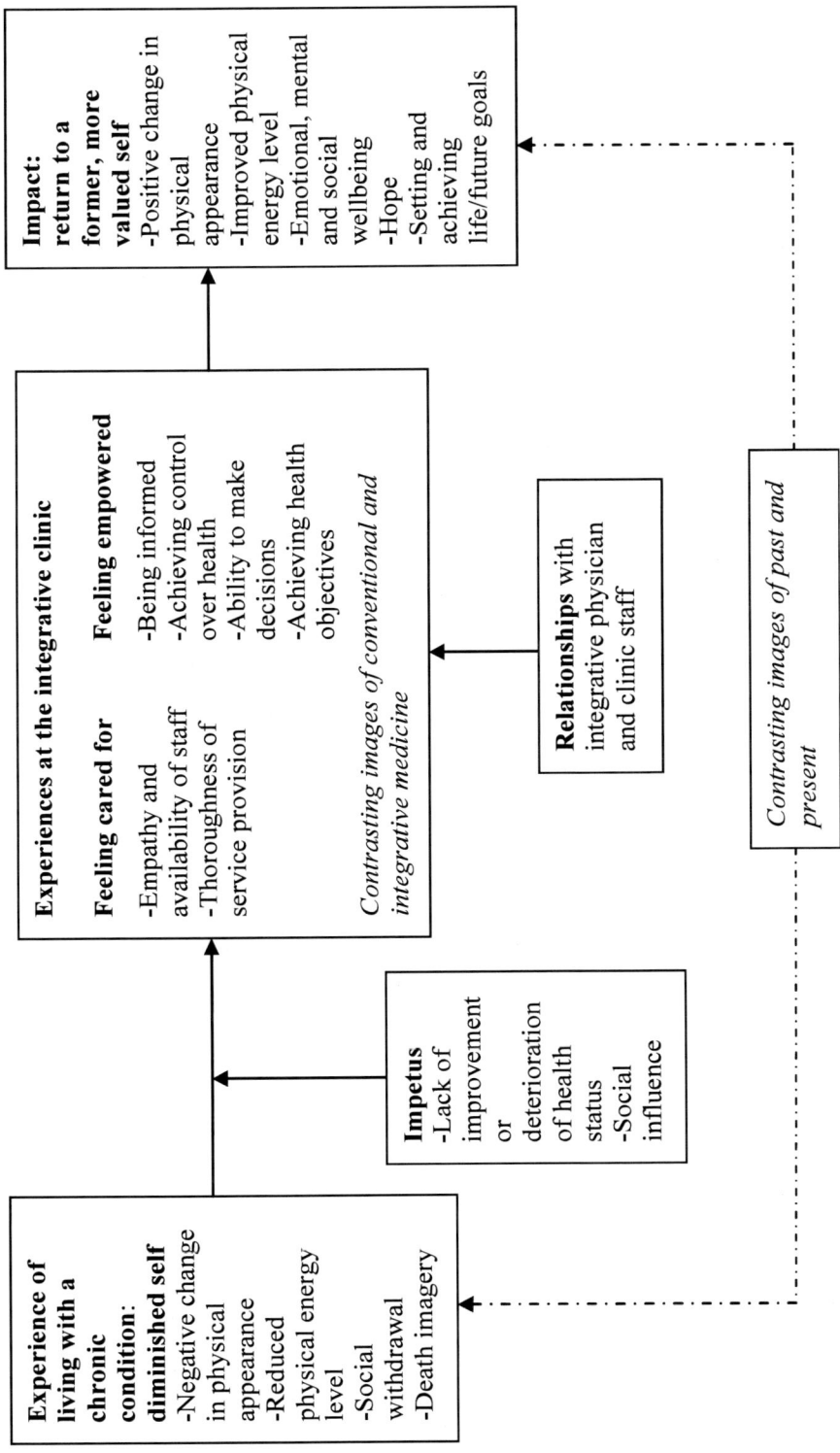

Figure 1. Participants' experiences of health conditions and relationships with caregivers.

I've gotten in trouble a lot because of lack of energy, like well why didn't you do this or that. Well I can't... I have three kids... and four grandchildren so I haven't been able to do much with them.

Withdrawal due to physical restrictions was also voiced by Adam. He did not have the patience to maintain social relationships and decried the quality of life he was leading.

Terrible, terrible life. No energy, no self... You lose the pride to life, you lose the ... joy of life... . Everything is a chore and when it comes to the end of the day, you say to... people, don't call me anymore please, lose my phone number.

The sense of loss, of having to forego enjoyable activities, was also evident in the participants' experiences of their illness. Marc pointed out:

I had to give up a lot of things... like chasing women was one of the things that just broke my heart... The hardest time of the year for me is winter, it's cold and windy. I can't go for a walk. It's maybe okay if you're healthy but trying to go for a walk when you're like me... When you sit around all winter long... it gets to you after a while... I don't have much of a personal life.

For some, death appeared as a better outcome than living with the illness as illustrated in Marc's account:

There are worse things in this world than dying... To live life when you... can't get around. What good is quality of life like that?

Participants' Initial Impetus to Join the Clinic

Participants indicated that the impetus to join the clinic was a health condition that was deteriorating or not improving, the lack of conventional treatment, and/or the influence of someone in the social milieu. Several participants described concerns or frustrations because their health was not improving even though they were following the required treatment regimen prescribed in the context of conventional medicine. Michael's account illustrates this concern:

Over a period of time I realized that... instead of the medication maintaining [my blood pressure] at what is considered an optimum level, 120 over 80, it started escalating... That concerned me. I'm taking what is supposed to maintain it at a proper level and instead of it staying there, over time it started escalating.

For a few participants, the integrative treatments offered at the clinic were seen as the last resort to improve their health. This was the case for Marc:

This is the only alternative I had. I can't go back to surgery. I'm toast there. I was in a clinical study... and that got stopped in a hurry because it was deemed to be cancer causing... So this is why I'm here.

Another impetus for seeking integrative care mentioned by participants was due to family or friends' suggestions. In the case of David, his son, a medical doctor, reinforced his decision to seek care at the clinic:

> I have a son who's a doctor... and I brought my son with me. And we sat down with Dr. Smith and we chatted for a long time, I mean Dr. Smith spent more time with my son than he did with me, ... explaining the protocol and the rationale ... behind what he was doing. And afterwards we went away and my son said, "Absolutely do it." And so that's how I got started.

One of Marc's impetuses for seeking health improvements was the influence of his golf "buddies":

> My buddies - I was in my hospital room, I was in pretty bad shape - came in and they said to me:...The guys at the golf course got together and we paid your membership this year... I thought to myself, I can't let them down. I've got to get better.

Relationships with Clinic Staff and the Impact on Participants' Experiences

Two major themes emerged from participants' accounts of their relationships with the integrative clinic staff and the impact these relationships had on their experience of their health condition: *feeling cared for* and *experiencing empowerment.*

Feeling Cared for

Participants expressed an appreciation for the clinic staff's empathy, availability, and thoroughness in their dealings with patients; this made participants feel that they were being cared for. Participants indicated that efforts to deliver patient oriented care started with the integrative physician. As Andre explained:

> I see the [staff members] here that I interact with as following in Dr. Smith's footsteps, by way of being, of caring, very knowledgeable and interested in helping you... It's so personal and directed towards you as the patient

Robert appreciated that staff always remembered the last conversation they had had with him.

> They see so many patients and they still remember what the conversation was last time you were here and I find that amazing.

Participants viewed the empathy, attention and care shown by providers as staff's interest in patients' life story and an attempt to build a meaningful rapport:

> Instead of a doctor-patient relationship it's more like a human to human relationship (Marc).

This helped to reaffirm participants' sense of self. This experience contrasts with what participants described as occurring in some conventional medicine clinics:

> The other places you're a statistic, a number, and you're almost made to feel you're lucky to get in... I'm certainly not impressed with... the level of care... It's less personal. (David).

The time restriction in conventional clinics was a particularly negative experience to participants. They experienced the thoroughness and the time dedicated by the providers at the integrative clinic as a further indication of care for the patients and their wellbeing:

> Dr. Smith just goes over everything, he writes it down on a piece of paper. He addresses each issue as you go along and then he asks questions to see if you have any other problems... And he's just very thorough... The last time I was at my doctor's, I was supposed to go in for a flu shot and she forgot all about it. (Allan).

Experiencing Empowerment

In addition to feeling cared for, participants experienced empowerment as a result of having more information on their health condition and of trying different healing modalities. Participants invariably viewed the integrative clinic providers as knowledgeable and helpful with sharing pertinent health information. Cynthia stated:

> Dr. Smith has a great way of explaining things in very simple terms. He's excellent at sharing knowledge.

Participants connected the information obtained from the staff to a better understanding of their condition, and to the ability to exert control over their health and life:

> When you sit down the first session, you really have to go home and do your homework. It's like a piano lesson, he gives you the work to take home and get better at it. So I took it home and ... tried to make myself better informed... And as you become more informed you become a better patient. And I think as you become a better patient... I actually feel like I have some control over my life. (Marc)

The experience was one of not only achieving a higher level of understanding and exerting more control, but also being in a position to make informed decisions:

> If you had a condition he gave you books to read on, websites to go to. He wanted to ensure that you were also educated on what your symptoms were, so that you can make the choices... I feel more empowered. I'm more trusting of what his recommendations are too. (Cynthia)

Here again, the participants resorted to comparisons between experiences in the integrative clinic and in other clinics, as illustrated by Marc:

> If you need to get more information, they tell you how to get it. I just feel like I'm part of the programme here as opposed to [conventional clinics].

The participants' experience at the integrative clinic also involved achieving health objectives that may not have been attainable in other medical contexts. Participants referred to the physician's ability to think outside the box, to combine Eastern and Western medicine, and to utilize different healing approaches. David's objectives included moving away from taking prescription medication that, he believed, was "treating symptoms rather than underlying causes and not with necessarily great outcomes":

You just knew you had to do something to get control and find some other alternative other than more pills and more pills and more pills... If you ask Dr. Smith something..., he will try to address it and he'll find natural ways to do it.

Participants' Experiences Following Treatment at the Integrative Clinic

Participants spoke about a number of experiences following treatments at the integrative clinic that included improvements at the physical, emotional and social levels of their lives, a return to a past self that was healthier, and having hope for or setting objectives for the future. Most participants spoke about noticing clear changes in their health condition, and the amount of change noticed depended on the severity of the patient's chronic illness.

Adam reported experiencing significant physical changes. The state of his feet were of particular concern to him because, as a diabetic patient, any further health deteriorations might have forced him to undergo an amputation. As someone in the construction business, he was required to be on his feet for long periods of time.

When I came here I had lost skin on one of my toes, my big toe was so dead I could take a needle, prick it, and I wouldn't feel it. Now, the health is back in my feet. I can walk without pain in my feet, without pain in my legs. I can last... I'm a contractor... can have a 16 hour day.

Marc's account is explicit about better mental health, clear in his reference to lack of depression, and experiencing spring fever, which he had not felt for 20 years:

I don't seem to be depressed. This was one of the best winters I've ever had as far as depression goes... I feel better generally... I feel younger. Because I haven't had spring fever for about 20 years. This spring I'm really feeling it.

Although Robert had not detected a change in his health status, he believed,

That's not a bad thing because I haven't noticed any deterioration either.

The experience of gaining control over one's health condition was also common, and related to this, was the management of medication. Daniel described the reduction of prescription medication:

It's also... gotten me off of a lot of drugs the regular doctors were prescribing to me. So I've cut down from all they were giving... but the ones for the diabetes.

Reducing the intake of prescription medication was not the only goal that participants had achieved. All participants expressed a desire to attain future health goals, which were revised as improvement in health was being experienced. Marc had an expectation of a longer life and was looking forward to going back to the golf course with his buddies:

So I'm in the programme here and I'm going to feel better. And I'm going to live long enough to get my old age pension cheque. And then I'll feel much, much better... As far as the social life goes, I'm looking forward to the golf season so that I can get out there with my buddies. Not have angina and not be worried every time I go out on the golf course whether it's my last trip.

David stated that he wanted to keep improving his health in order to spend more time with his grandchildren.

> I've got seven grandchildren and I thought to myself, I got to be around, I want to see these kids grow up, because we had so much fun with our own growing up and whatnot. So I just wanted to feel healthy, I wanted to be active.

The importance of participants' social connections was obvious not only in their reflections on their goals for better health, but also in terms of confirmation that better health had been achieved. Participants reported that changes to their health since beginning treatments had been noticed by others around them, and this served as an encouragement to continue their treatments. Cynthia remarked on the reaction of her family and colleagues:

> Everyone actually has a made a comment... They notice a big difference in me... They just say you look great. Keep it up.

David indicated that improvements in his health condition were confirmed not only by his family members, but also by his endocrinologist.

> My last visit to the endocrinologist, I was going every three months. She said, I don't need to see you for six months. It was normal. So to me that's a good measurement, things are working.

DISCUSSION

There are strong contrasts between participants' accounts of experiences of health condition before starting treatment at the integrative clinic and after receiving treatment. The restoration of physical characteristics, energy levels, physical and social activities, and emotional and mental states experienced in earlier stages of life signal a return to a more valued self – one that was lost due to the chronic illness. A fixation with death for some participants, prevalent in accounts before undertaking integrative medicine treatments were replaced by images of hope, expectations and future-oriented goals.

The negative accounts of participants' experiences before seeking treatment are consistent with Charmaz's (1983) and Bury's (1982) research showing that chronic illness threatens the individual self and biography. Participants' inability to fulfill roles and activities that defined them in the past poses a threat to self. Charmaz indicates that "chronically ill patients frequently experience a crumbling away of their former self-images without simultaneous development of equally valued new ones" (1983:168). She further states that these individuals experience their developing limitations as losses. The loss theme is clear in participants' accounts; it is evident in contrasts that the participants made between the present and the past states. Much of the experience of suffering and loss of self is based on "the inability to control one's self and life in ways that had been hoped for, anticipated or assumed" (Charmaz, 1983:187). Chronic illness encroaches upon life, eroding people's selves as well as their health (Charmaz, 1995). The notion of possible selves proposed by Markus and Nurius (1986) is pertinent here. They point out that "possible selves represent individuals' ideas of what they may become, what they would like to become, and what they are afraid of becoming" (1986:954). Possible selves "function as incentives for future behaviour (i.e. they are selves to be approached or avoided)" and "provide an evaluative and interpretive context for the current view of self" (1986:954). In participants' accounts, a new self was made possible through active participation in healing following from attending the integrative medicine clinic.

There is a strong contrast in the experiences related by participants before and after seeking treatment at the integrative clinic. Images of hair growing back, ability to work long hours again, and establishing control over health conditions contrast strongly with the images that participants provided of their experience prior to integrative treatments. Having hope and setting goals for the future – such as collecting pension payments and having fun with grandchildren – provide a strong contrast to the negative perspectives before receiving treatments. For some, there is a return to an earlier past – or an earlier self – that was experienced before the debilitating effects of illness set in. In other words, there is a re-entering of the worlds they left earlier (Charmaz, 1995). The experiences post integrative treatments are cast vis-a-vis two different pasts that are used as frames for seeing the self – the past preceding the onset of illness (which is valued) and the past where the suffering from the illness was experienced (which is devalued).

The discrepancy between the participants' vision of desired health and their poorly perceived health status, the experience of the limits of conventional approaches, and the influence of others in the social milieu provided impetus to seek alternative treatment modalities. These elements are consistent with Markus and Nurius' (1986) argument that a discrepancy between the desired self and the current self provides incentives for behaviours, and with Ohlen et al.'s (2006) finding that significant others have an important influence on patients' treatment decision making.

Participants' relationships and care received at the integrative clinic were experienced against the backdrop of their previous encounters in the context of conventional medicine. Here again, contrast is a central element in the participants' experiences. Past experience of limited time with health care providers, dealing with localized health problems, having little information on one's health condition, and experiencing the side effects of medication provided a context for participants' reflections on the relationships and the care they received at the integrative clinic. Experiences at the clinic referred to empathy, availability of time, thoroughness, information sharing, holistic approaches, diversity of treatment modalities, empowerment, and ability to exert control over one's health and life.

The importance of relationships and communications between patients and health care providers in terms of patient well-being and satisfaction and/or health improvement has been well documented in the literature (e.g. Allen et al., 2011; Brown, 2008; Skirbekk et al., 2011; S.K. Smith et al., 2009). Our findings show that patients look for empathy and thorough attention from health care providers to their health problems. There were comparisons between some conventional medicine contexts in which patients were made to feel like "a statistic, a number", a drain on time and resources, and the integrative clinic where providers give ample time and the physician "goes over everything". This is similar to Allen et al.'s (2011) finding that patients contrast whole person care with "assembly line" treatment, and that their trust in health professionals is tied to the ability of the latter to listen to patients and integrate their explanations in health management. The notion of trust in our findings was tied not only to the thoroughness shown by the providers, but also to their investment in educating patients about their conditions. As one of our participants stated, the physician's efforts in ensuring that the patient was educated on her illness allowed her to be more trusting of his recommendations, as well as to make choices and feel more empowered.

The patient-practitioner relationship (including trust) as well as the practitioner's communication skills influences patient involvement in health care decision making (S.K. Smith et al., 2009). Allen et al. (2011) emphasized the importance of the patient-clinician relationship for chronic illness management, pointing to the need to have joint decision-making that integrates the patients' experience with medical expertise. Our results are consistent with their findings that "patients want to be treated as whole persons and respected knowledgeable partners in the management of (chronic) illness which occurs and is experienced in not just a body, but in a unique life-world" (2011:134). This was clear in our participants' accounts of "human to human relationship" instead of a doctor-patient relationship, and in their mentioning that they felt they had time to tell their illness story to attentive and empathetic health care providers.

CONCLUSION

In this paper we have attended to chronically ill patients' experiences of deteriorating health, seeking integrative medicine treatments and experiencing health improvements. We have attended to the sense of self in situations of deteriorating and improving health, drawing attention to the contrasts that chronically ill patients make between past and present, loss and hope, impoverished and empowering relationships with care providers, and conventional and integrative treatments.

It would be a mistake to conclude from this study that conventional medicine comes with so many limitations that alternative or integrative approaches are able to overcome. Although this may have been the experience of our participants, it should be remembered that our study relied on a small sample of individuals who received treatment at an integrative clinic. Another limitation of our study is that individuals self selected for participation in the study. They all reported experiencing positive health effects. We do not know the extent to which chronically ill patients who join similar integrative programs achieve positive health outcomes. This is an issue that can be investigated in a different type of study. Yet some of the experiences that we report are consistent with findings from other studies, and more importantly, are revealing of what some patients with chronic illness experience when their health deteriorates and then improves following the use of more holistic approaches. An important element in experiencing a healthier body and self was the relationship that patients established with providers and the type of care they received.

Numerous studies have appeared over the years on the importance of provider-patient relationship and communication (Aujoulat et al., 2007; Kim et al., 2004; Maizes et al., 2009; McCaffrey et al., 2007; Mead & Bower, 2000; Scott et al., 2008; Squier, 1990). Study after study has argued for or shown the importance of providing patient centered care, and empowering patients by giving them a voice and providing them with education and tools to manage their illness. As our findings have shown, having some control over one's health and achieving better health outcomes go a long way in establishing a sense of self-worth and living a more fulfilling life. Brown (2008) has argued that a paternal model of interaction where the physician is seen to possess expert knowledge and the patient is precluded from treatment decisions has become less viable. "Power in the 'new' patient-professional relationship has been redistributed and is much less asymmetric... Consequently, the professional's standing as caring and competent is now likely to depend to a greater degree on involving the patient" (Brown, 2008:357).

As a growing segment of the population age, and the increasing occurrence of chronic illness becomes more likely, there is a need for serious thinking on the part of policy makers, professional associations and institutions involved in the education of health providers to consider the changes necessary to bring about and institute new frames and practices. We refer specifically to frames and practices that would allow providers to offer the type of care that values patients as individuals with unique health stories and provides them with the tools to control and manage their illness. As Allen et al. indicate, "In no other context is patient collaboration more important than in the ongoing management of chronic illness and disease where patients' daily self-care can be in harmony or in conflict with health professionals' medical interventions" (2011:133).

At a systematic level, chronic illnesses such as heart disease, diabetes and asthma impose a significant burden on the health care system. For example, in Canada, where this study was conducted, costs incurred in order to treat chronic ailments account for 55 percent of all health care costs (Tsasis & Bains, 2008). Individuals with chronic illnesses use homecare and hospital services to a greater extent than other patients (Broemeling et al., 2008). The present health care structure is built to address acute rather than chronic care needs—with greater emphasis placed on treating the immediate (and urgent) needs than on disease management and prevention (Bodenheimer et al., 2002). As a result of this structure, most patients suffering from chronic conditions do not receive the resources or the time necessary to properly manage their condition, and as such, receive substandard care (Bodenheimer *et al.*, 2002).

In conclusion, we believe that micro level studies – such as ours – that give insight into the lived experience of chronic illness need to be complemented by macro level studies that offer systems level analysis of structures, incentive systems, and educational/training programs for providers. For example, there is a need to consider how incentives can be worked into the system that would allow providers to dedicate more time to chronically ill patients. Until more lasting and broad-based changes occur in health provision modalities – which currently tend towards limiting time and contact with the patient – studies of lived experience will continue to report on the suffering of those who have illnesses and feel they have to contend with impoverished selves and lives.

REFERENCES

Allen, D., Wainwright, M., & Hutchinson, T. (2011). 'Non-compliance' as illness management: Hemodialysis patients' descriptions of adversarial patient-clinician interactions. *Social Science & Medicine, 73*, 129-134.,

Aujoulat, I., d'Hoore, W., & Deccache, A. (2007). Patient empowerment in theory and practice: Polysemy or cacophony? *Patient Education and Counseling, 66*(1), 13-20.

Baumeister, R.F. (1997). Identity, self-concept, and self-esteem: The self lost and found. In Hogan, R., Johnson, J., & Briggs, S. (Eds.), *Handbook of personality psychology,* San Diego: Academic Press, 681-710.

Bell, I. R., Caspi, O., Schwartz, G. E., Grant, K. L., Gaudet, T. W., Rychener, D., et al. (2002). Integrative medicine and systemic outcomes research: Issues in the emergence of a new model for primary health care. *Archives of Internal Medicine, 162*(2), 133-140.

Bodenheimer, T., Lorig, K., Holman, H., & Grumbach, K. (2002). Patient self-management of chronic disease in primary care. *Journal of the American Medical Association, 288*(19), 2469-2475.

Bodenheimer, T., Wagner, E. H., & Grumbach, K. (2002). Improving primary care for patients with chronic illness. *Journal of the American Medical Association, 288*(14), 1775-1779.

Broemeling, A. M., Watson, D. E., & Prebtani, F. (2008). Population patterns of chronic health conditions, co-morbidity and healthcare use in canada: Implications for policy and practice. *Healthcare Quarterly, 11*(3), 70-76.

Brown, P.R. (2008). Trusting in the new NHS: instrumental versus communicative action. *Sociology of Health & Illness, 30,* 349-363.

Bury, M. (1982). Chronic illness as biographical disruption. *Sociology of Health and Illness, 4*(2), 167-182.

Clare, L. (2003). Managing threats to self: awareness in early stage Alzheimer's disease. *Social Science & Medicine,57,*1017-1029

Charmaz, K. (1983). Loss of self: A fundamental form of suffering in the chronically ill. *Sociology of Health and Illness, 5*(2), 168-195.

Charmaz, K. (1995). The body, identity, and self: adapting to impairment. *The Sociological Quarterly, 36,* 657-680.

Creswell, J.W. (2007). *Qualitative inquiry and research design: Choosing among five approaches, 2nd ed.* Thousand Oaks, CA: Sage.

Fuertes, J. N., Mislowack, A., Bennett, J., Paul, L., Gilbert, T. C., Fontan, G., et al. (2007). The physician-patient working alliance. *Patient Education and Counseling, 66*(1), 29-36.

Goldring, A. B., Taylora, S. E., Kemeny, M. E., & Anton, P. A. (2002). Impact of health beliefs, quality of life, and the physician-patient relationship on the treatment intentions of inflammatory bowel disease patients. *Health Psychology, 21*(3), 219-228.

Haugli, L., Strand, E., & Finset, A. (2004). How do patients with rheumatic disease experience their relationship with their doctors? A qualitative study of experiences of stress and support in the doctor-patient relationship. *Patient Education and Counseling, 52*(2), 169-174.

Hok, J., Wachtler, C., Falkenberg, T., & Tishelman, C. (2007). Using narrative analysis to understand the combined use of complementary therapies and bio-medically oriented health care. *Social Science & Medicine, 65,* 1642-1653.

Horowitz, C. R., Rein, S. B., & Leventhal, H. (2004). A story of maladies, misconceptions and mishaps: Effective management of heart failure. *Social Science and Medicine, 58*(3), 631-643.

Ironside, P.M., Schekel, M., Wessels, C., Powers, S, & Seeley, D.K. (2003). Experiencing chronic illness: cocreating new understandings. *Qualitative Health Research, 13* 171-183.

Kaplan, S. H., Greenfield, S., & Ware Jr., J. E. (1989). Assessing the effects of physician-patient interactions on the outcomes of chronic disease. *Medical Care, 27*(3 Suppl), S110-127.

Kim, S. S., Kaplowitz, S., & Johnston, M. V. (2004). The effects of physician empathy on patient satisfaction and compliance. *Evaluation and the Health Professions, 27*(3), 237-251.

Koithan, M., Bell, I. R., Caspi, O., Ferro, L., & Brown, V. (2007). Patients' experiences and perceptions of a consultative model integrative medicine clinic: A qualitative study. *Integrative Cancer Therapies, 6*(2), 174-184.

Maizes, V., Rakel, D., & Niemiec, C. (2009). Integrative medicine and patient-centered care. *EXPLORE: The Journal of Science and Healing, 5*(5), 277-289.

Markus, H., & Nurius, P. (1986). Possible selves. *American Psychologist, 4*, 1954-969.

McCaffrey, A. M., Pugh, G. F., & O'Connor, B. B. (2007). Understanding patient preference for integrative medical care: Results from patient focus groups. *Journal of General Internal Medicine: Official Journal of the Society for Research and Education in Primary Care Internal Medicine, 22*(11), 1500-1505.

Mead, N., & Bower, P. (2000). Patient-centredness: A conceptual framework and review of the empirical literature. *Social Science and Medicine, 51*(7), 1087-1110.

Miles, M. B., & A. Michael Huberman. (1994). In Holland R. (Ed.), *An expanded sourcebook: Qualitative data analysis* (2nd ed.). Thousand Oaks, California: Sage Publications.

Ohlen, J., Balneaves, L.G., Bottorff, J.L., & Brazier, A.S.A. (2006). The influence of significant others in complementary and alternative medicine decisions by cancer patients. *Social Science & Medicine, 63*, 1625-1636.

Öhman, M., Söderberg, S., & Lundman, B. (2003). Hovering between suffering and enduring: The meaning of living with serious chronic illness. *Qualitative Health Research, 13*(4), 528-542.

Parchman, M. L., Noel, P. H., & Lee, S. (2005). Primary care attributes, health care system hassles, and chronic illness. *Medical Care, 43*(11), 1123-1129.

Raheim, M., & Haland. W. (2003). Lived experience of chronic pain and fibromyalgia: Women's stories from daily life. *Qualitative Health Research, 16*, 741-761.

Scott, J. G., Cohen, D., DiCicco-Bloom, B., Miller, W. L., Stange, K. C., & Crabtree, B. F. (2008). Understanding healing relationships in primary care. *Annals of Family Medicine, 6*(4), 315-322.

Skirbekk, H., Middelthon, A-L., Hjortdahl, P., & Finset, A. (2011). Mandates of trust in the doctor-patient relationship. *Qualitative Health Research, 21*, 1182-1190.

Smith, J.A., Flowers, P., & Larkin, M. (2009). *Interpretative phenomenological analysis.* London: Sage Publications.

Smith, L., Bosnic-Anticevich, S. Z., Mitchell, B., Saini, B., Krass, I., & Armour, C. (2007). Treating asthma with a self-management model of illness behaviour in an Australian community pharmacy setting. *Social Science and Medicine, 64*(7), 1501-1511.

Smith, S.K., Dixon, A., Trevena, L., Nutbeam, D., & McCaffery, K.J. (2009). Exploring patient involvement in healthcare decision making across different education and functional health literacy groups. *Social Science & Medicine, 69*, 1805-1812.

Stake, R.E. (1995). *The art of case study research.* Thousand Oaks, CA: Sage.

Squier, R. (1990). A model of empathic understanding and adherence to treatment regimens in practitioner-patient relationships. *Social Science and Medicine, 30*(3), 325-339.

Tsasis, P., & Bains, J. (2008). Management of complex chronic disease: Facing the challenges in the Canadian health-care system. *Health Services Management Research : An Official Journal of the Association of University Programs in Health Administration / HSMC, AUPHA, 21*(4), 228-235.

Wasson, J. H., Johnson, D. J., Benjamin, R., Phillips, J., & MacKenzie, T. A. (2006). Patients report positive impacts of collaborative care. *Journal of Ambulatory Care Management, 29*(3), 199-206.

Whittemore, R., & Dixon, J. (2008). Chronic illness: The process of integration. *Journal of Clinical Nursing, 17*(7B), 177-187.

Yin, R.K. (2003). *Case study research: Design and methods*, (3rd ed.). Thousand Oaks, CA: Sage.

In: Alternative Medicine
Editors: Kenneth R. Carter and George E. Murphy

ISBN 978-1-62257-106-2
©2012 Nova Science Publishers, Inc.

Chapter 5

COMPLEMENTARY AND ALTERNATIVE MEDICINE USE IN CHILDREN WITH INFLAMMATORY BOWEL DISEASE

Andrew S. Day and Stephen J. Robinson*
Department of Paediatrics, University of Otago (Christchurch),
Christchurch, New Zealand

ABSTRACT

Following diagnosis with a chronic incurable illness, such as Inflammatory Bowel Disease (IBD), children and their families often face uncertainty and worries.

These include concerns about the need for standard medical therapies, and the potential side-effects of these treatments. Further, the available drugs have variable benefits and may not always assist adequately in the management of the child's disease.

Consequently, many parents and families look to other options, including complementary and alternative medicines (CAM) as ways to help their child's condition.

INTRODUCTION

Complementary and Alternative medicines (CAM) include a variety of types and modalities of therapies.[1, 2] A number of these interventions are considered to have specific benefits for the gastrointestinal (GI) tract, such as enhancement of gut function, modulation of host-pathogen interactions and improvement of symptoms related to the gut. Probiotics, organisms that induce a beneficial effect after ingestion, are one example of a CAM that may have such effects. In addition, other CAM interventions may improve the individual's general well-being or enhance the person's abilities to cope with stressful events. Such potential benefits may be especially relevant for someone suffering with a chronic illness.

* Phone: 64-3-3640-747, Fax: 64-3-3640919, Email : andrew.day@otago.ac.nz.

Inflammatory bowel disease is an example of a chronic illness affecting the GI tract, leading to bowel and systemic symptoms and consequences. [3] Consequently, CAM agents could be considered to have roles in the ongoing management of this condition. In addition, CAM usage tends to be higher in individuals with chronic, debilitating or life threatening illnesses. In one study, for instance, three times as many children with IBD or cerebral palsy were using CAM than healthy children. [4]

This chapter will highlight important features of IBD in childhood, review recent data on the patterns of use of CAM in this patient group and consider key aspects of this practice.

INFLAMMATORY BOWEL DISEASE

Crohn Disease and Ulcerative Colitis

The condition known as Inflammatory Bowel Disease (IBD) encompasses two main diseases: Crohn disease (CD) and Ulcerative colitis (UC). [3] These types of IBD can be differentiated by disease distribution within the gut, inflammatory patterns and specific histologic features. [3,5] CD can affect any section of the gastrointestinal tract (GIT), involves transmural inflammation and features granulomata. UC on the other hand involves the colon, for a variable distance from the rectum, with superficial inflammation prominent. Some individuals will have features of IBD, but without features that distinguish between CD and UC: this is termed IBD Unclassified (IBDU).

Both CD and UC can be seen as incurable, and both have a relapsing-remitting course over the lifetime of the patient. Recent large series have demonstrated that the patterns of CD and UC differ between children and adults. [6, 7] Paediatric-onset UC, for instance, is predominantly pan-colonic with proctitis alone being uncommon. Further, those children with more localised involvement at diagnosis often have extension of disease over the first years after diagnosis. In paediatric CD, upper gut involvement occurs in up to two thirds of children, but less than 10% of adults. [6]

Although the precise causes of IBD have not yet been defined, it is commonly accepted that IBD occurs as a result of interactions between the intestinal mucosa and the luminal contents (especially the intestinal microflora or their byproducts), which lead to dysregulated inflammation in a genetically susceptible host. Over the last few decades, rates of IBD have increased in many countries, especially in European countries. [8] High rates of CD have been noted in Australasia since the turn of the century. [9, 10] Furthermore, in the recent years, increasing rates have been seen in additional parts of the world, especially in Asian countries where IBD was thought to be most uncommon. [11]

Both CD and UC can begin at any age. Around a quarter of individuals develop features of IBD in childhood – with increasing rates seen from infancy to the highest rates in adolescent years. [12] When diagnosed in children, CD and UC have huge potential adverse impacts upon growth, pubertal development, and daily activities.

Nutritional and Other Consequences of IBD in Children

Almost all children with CD, and up to two thirds of those with UC, have a history of weight loss or poor weight gain at the time of diagnosis. [13] Furthermore, many children will have altered linear growth and some will have delayed pubertal development at diagnosis. Following diagnosis, a number of children will have ongoing problems with growth, and pubertal development. The latter is especially a problem in boys with their pubertal period starting later and extending for a longer time. [14]

Growth disruption is consequent partly to impaired dietary intake, but especially to uncontrolled inflammation. The pro-inflammatory cytokine, interleukin (IL)-6 impairs synthesis and activity of insulin-like growth factor (IGF)-1, a key signalling component of the growth hormone (GH) pathway. [15] In addition, IL-6 and tumour-necrosis-factor (TNF)-α also adversely impact growth plate function. [15]

In addition, CD and UC commonly adversely affect the day to day functioning of children or adolescents with these conditions. [16] This may include interruption to schooling, inability to perform sports or difficulty with socialisation.

Further, depression and anxiety occur at higher rates. These aspects can be considered as components of health related quality of life (QOL). QOL in children and adolescents with IBD can be assessed using a specific tool (IMPACT questionnaire) that was developed and validated for the context of paediatric IBD. [17] This device has been translated and adapted for several different countries.

Management of IBD in Childhood

Whilst one goal of the management of IBD in children is to resolve inflammation (and related symptoms), broader objectives include maintaining normal growth and development, and ensuring optimal quality of day to day functioning.

Standard therapies include drugs, nutritional interventions and surgical procedures. Some of these are administered as short-term agents to reduce inflammation (i.e. to induce disease remission). Others are provided as longer-term maintenance therapies (i.e. to prevent relapse). However, none of the available therapies for paediatric CD are curative. In addition, almost all therapies have potential side-effects. Hence, the benefits of a therapy need to be weighed against the potential adverse effects of this intervention within the individual patient context. Almost all children and adolescents will commence a therapy following diagnosis and will have ongoing therapies throughout childhood. Many children will take a number of medicines over each day. Despite these interventions, these children remain at risk of relapse of disease (which may be triggered by stress-full events or consequent to inter-current infections).

Consequent to the persistent and pervasive features of CD and UC in childhood, and in the context of no curable intervention, the parents of many children consider other options, including complementary and alternative medicines (CAM). The use of CAM therapies, the range of available agents and contributory factors have been evaluated in a number of studies over the last decade.

USE OF CAM IN IBD

CAM Therapies Considered for IBD

A range of CAM therapies have been considered and may have relevance for individuals with IBD. [2] Some CAM therapies may have direct anti-inflammatory effects that could enhance disease control in conjunction with standard treatments. These include nutritional interventions, agents that may enhance host immune responses and interventions that may modulate psychological or emotional responses to the disease. Herbal therapies appear to be the most commonly used CAM, but variations occur between cultures and regions of the world.

Langmead and Rampton [2] reviewed the data supporting particular CAM therapies in the context of IBD. The principal conclusions of this review were that there is little controlled data regarding agents that have been commonly suggested for IBD. Note was made, however, of promising data arising from studies examining acupuncture in IBD. Hillsden and colleagues [18] made a similar statement regarding the evidence supporting CAM in IBD and referred to specific resources, including internet databases of available CAM agents.

CAM Usage in Adults with IBD

A series of studies conducted in Canada late last century demonstrated some key features of CAM use in adults with IBD. An initial study was conducted in a group of 134 adults with IBD (mostly CD) using a structured questionnaire. [19] Fifty-one percent of this group had used CAM agents in the preceding 24 months, whilst one third of the cohort was currently taking a CAM. In the current user group, half had introduced a CAM specifically for their IBD, whilst the others were using them for different indications. Disease duration and hospitalization were associated directly with the current use of CAM. Concerns about standard medical therapies (either side-effects and/or lack of efficacy) were commonly stated by the respondents.

The same group of investigators subsequently used an internet-based approach to ascertain the CAM usage patterns in a wider group of subjects. [20] Two hundred and sixty-three adults completed the web-based questionnaire. Almost half of this group (46%) had utilised CAM agents in the previous 2 years, with current use reported by 34%. Again, similar to the clinic-based cohort, these adults were most commonly using herbal products, vitamins and natural health products and they reported use of CAM because of concerns about adverse effects or ineffectiveness of standard medical therapies.

These investigators also evaluated reasons for the use of CAM in patients with IBD using a multi-method approach in a smaller group of adults. [21] Fourteen patients underwent in-depth interviews to elucidate usage patterns and their reasons for choice of CAM agent. As noted in the questionnaire-based group, dissatisfaction with standard medical care and concerns about side-effects were commonly seen. The patients generally felt that CAM agents were safe and reported a number of reasons for not discussing their choice with their own medical practitioner.

Rawsthorne and colleagues assessed usage in adults with IBD from four distinct centres located in USA, Ireland, Canada and Sweden. [22] Two hundred and eighteen patients were included and all completed a self-administered questionnaire. Rates of CAM use varied between 31% and 68%, with higher rates seen in North American patients. The most common CAM modalities in this series were exercise, prayer, counselling, massage, chiropractic and relaxation therapies. Factors supporting the respondents' use of CAM included satisfaction with standard therapies, unfavourable attitude to healthcare facilities, and sense of hopelessness about their medical state.

A British study conducted earlier this century focused more on the relationships between QOL and CAM usage. [23] A population of 239 adults completed questionnaires about CAM use and completed a validated QOL tool. Overall, 26% of this group utilised CAM for their disease. QOL scores for fatigue, anxiety and malaise dimensions were lower in CAM users than in non-users. Overall QOL scores were not different between the two groups however. Furthermore, multivariate analysis indicated that fatigue was the only variable still associated with CAM use.

A more recent report from the UK documented current or previous usage by 39% of a group of 160 adults with known IBD. [24] Vitamins and herbal products were most commonly utilised. These individuals received advice about the selection of CAM from a variety of sources, including health professionals.

The use of CAM in adults with IBD was reviewed systematically recently, with focus upon reports that included 100 or more adult subjects with IBD. [18] Overall, rates of current use of CAM across these studies ranged from 11 to 34%, with rates of past or current use as high as 60%. A range of factors for the use of CAM were identified, with these being dependent upon the situation and methodology used to collect data. Overall, however, common factors include disease severity and duration, requirements for standard medications, quality of life, history of surgical intervention and requirement for hospitalisation.

USE OF CAM IN CHILDREN AND ADOLESCENTS WITH IBD

A number of studies have examined the usage of CAM by children and adolescents with IBD. Although some similar patterns have been observed, there are also regional and/or cultural differences in use. Further, there are some key aspects that differ from CAM patterns in adults diagnosed with IBD.

In general, the decision to administer CAM therapies to children and adolescents will likely be made by a parent or caregiver, rather than the individual child themselves. Consequently, the decision making process may reflect parental attitudes along with perceived requirements and responses.

We have examined CAM usage in Australian children attending gastroenterology clinics [25, 26] and attending specific IBD clinics. [27] More than one third of 92 children attending a range of gastroenterology clinics were being administered CAM in an initial questionnaire-based study.[25] Just 10 of this group had been diagnosed with IBD: three of these 10 children were taking CAM. Ninety percent of the parents of the 92 children reported that they would consider a CAM agent for their child if recommended.

A subsequent report a decade later involved 98 children attending general gastroenterology clinics in the same hospital (but none with IBD). [26] This report demonstrated increased recent or current usage (69%), with wide awareness and acceptance by parents. The children in this cohort were being managed for a variety of GI conditions, but none of the group were diagnosed with IBD.

In addition, a further questionnaire-based assessment solely of children diagnosed with IBD in the same hospital was conducted. [27] This report involved the responses from 46 families following receipt of a mailed questionnaire. Almost three quarters of the children were reported by their parents to be receiving CAM, which was more than double the rate of the children without IBD from the same location. On average these children were receiving 2.4 CAM agents, with four children having five or more therapies. Fish oil and probiotics were the most common agents utilised. Interestingly only 12% of the CAM-users reported the agents to be very effective – however 50% of the users also noted partial benefits. In this cohort, there were no associations between age, gender, disease type or duration of disease and CAM usage. [27]

In contrast to the high rates seen in this Australian group, much lower rates were seen in a Canadian cohort of children with IBD. [28] Twenty-two percent of this group reported having ever used CAM, whilst only 6.7% reported current use. Other European and North American reports have defined rates between these extremes.

Heuschkel and colleagues [29] surveyed 208 children between two centres in USA and one in the United Kingdom. CAM usage was reported in 41%, with megavitamins, diet supplements, and herbal remedies most commonly administered. Higher rates of CAM usage were seen in children whose parents also use CAM and those who had more adverse effects from standard drugs. Furthermore, 59% of non-users reported an interest in learning more about CAM.

A similar rate of CAM usage was determined in a large cohort of 334 children recruited from the greater Philadelphia area. [30] Although megavitamins were also used commonly, nutritional supplements, probiotics and fish oil were frequently reported. The factors associated with use of CAM were explored in more detail in this study. Univariate analysis suggested that CD, access to the internet, poor QOL and more frequent school absences were factors for the use of CAM. Further regression analysis ascertained that poor QOL, use of the internet for research and a need for calorie supplementation were all factors linked with use of CAM. In addition, those individuals requiring surgical procedures had lower rates of CAM use than those who the subjects who did not require surgery.

A different set of factors was illustrated in a recent report of the use of CAM in 86 Scottish children. [31] A higher number of courses of steroids, more parental education and lower patient age were reported by the parents of these children as the key factors for the use of CAM. Around two thirds of the group had used and 37% were currently using, with probiotics and diaryfree diet being most commonly administered. However, 89% of the parents in this group reported that they would consider giving CAM in the future.

Probiotics were again reported as the most commonly utilised agent in a North American study involving 236 children with IBD within 3 separate sites. [32] In addition to the children with IBD, this study also recruited children with other chronic disease states. Half of the children with IBD included in this study used CAM, which was greater than rates of use seen in children with other chronic disease states. Educational achievement, general well-being,

European background, and a history of more side-effects from standard drugs were factors linked with CAM use in this group.

The use of Mind-Body CAM was examined recently in a group of 67 adolescents with IBD. [33] Mind-body CAMs include relaxation, meditation, prayer or similar modalities. In this cohort, prayer was used most commonly (62% of the group), with relaxation and imagery also used frequently. Younger age, more severe disease and worse QOL were all associated with increased willingness to consider using these CAM interventions.

Adolescents might be expected to make their own decisions regarding the use of CAM (rather than a parental decision), especially for mind-body modalities that require personal activity (such as praying). Decision making about the use of CAM in adolescent patients was explored in depth in a recently published case report. [34] One pertinent issue is regarding who has the authority to make a decision involving an adolescent – the adolescent or the parent.

Although decision making, whether by an adolescent themselves or by parent on behalf of their child, is one aspect of the use of CAM, another important aspect of the use of CAM therapies is clear communication about the use of these agents. It is important for practitioners to be able to introduce the concept of CAM usage within the therapeutic relationship, and also for the practitioner to remember to ask about possible usage. Furthermore, if asked about a CAM agent by a patient or parent, then the practitioner should endeavour to answer with an open and non-dismissive approach, in order to maintain clear lines of communication. One New Zealand study ascertained that only 11% of patients could recall having been asked by a doctor if they were using CAM. [35] Further, almost one quarter of the patients in our recent questionnaire-based study had not told their doctor about their use of CAM. [26] These data highlight the importance of communication in children with IBD who may be using CAM agents.

CONCLUSION

Overall, CAM agents are commonly administered to children with IBD. Most reports indicate that at least 40% of such children have recently been given CAM, with a smaller number currently using. Rates and the pattern of CAM agents administered differ between the reported studies, with variations within and between countries.

These differences may reflect methodological differences, with different questionnaires and different approaches to collected data evident. Standardisation of questionnaires and the adoption of consistent methods more generally would ensure more direct comparison between these groups. Even if such a standard approach was adopted, it is likely that variation between countries would persist, reflecting different cultural attitudes to CAM and different patterns of access to various CAM agents.

Furthermore, the available studies highlight differences in the factors reported to influence CAM usage between European and North American cohorts. Again these variations may reflect access to particular CAM agents.

Overall, the available data demonstrate much greater use of CAM in children with IBD, than in children with other GI conditions, or in well children. It is unclear if this is a reflection of the chronic and incurable nature of IBD, or the specific involvement of the GI tract (and consequent bowel symptoms). In addition, increasing rates of CAM usage in children with IBD may reflect changes and attitudes in the wider community.

Probiotics and fish oil are two widely used agents in children with IBD. This may reflect the wider exposure of information about these agents consequent to numerous scientific reports. Even though the data to universally support these therapies is lacking, the fact that these have been subject to scientific scrutiny may have enhanced their profile. Other agents with less awareness or exposure may be utilised less as a consequence.

In conclusion, CAM agents are used frequently by children and adolescents with IBD in almost every reported study. It is likely that rates will continue to increase. Paediatric gastroenterologists caring for children with IBD must ensure adequate personal understanding and awareness of CAM agents, and have a working knowledge of potential roles, possible interactions and contraindications. Furthermore, paediatric gastroenterologists must remember to ask patients and parents about their use of CAM.

REFERENCES

[1]   Kong SC, Hurlstone DP, Pocock CY, et al. The incidence of self-prescribed oral complementary and alternative medicine use by patients with gastrointestinal diseases. *J. Clin. Gastroenterol.* 2005; 39:138-141.

[2]   Langmead L, Rampton DS. Review article: complementary and alternative therapies for inflammatory bowel disease. *Aliment. Pharmacol. Ther.* 2006; 23: 341-9.

[3]   Griffiths AM, Hugot J-P. Crohn Disease. Chapter 41, Pediatric Gastrointestinal Disease, 4th Edition. Eds: Walker A, Goulet O, Kleinman RE, et al., BC Decker, Hamilton Ontario, 2004.

[4]   McCann LJ, Newell SJ. Survey of paediatric complementary and alternative medicine use in health and chronic illness. *Arch. Dis. Child.* 2006; 91: 173-4.

[5]   IBD Working Group of the European Society for Paediatric Gastroenterology, Hepatology and Nutrition. Inflammatory bowel disease in children and adolescents: Recommendations for diagnosis – The Porto criteria. *J. Pediatr. Gastroenterol. Nutr.* 2005;41: 1-7.

[6]   Van Limbergen J, Russell RK, Drummond HE, Aldhous MC, Round NK, Nimmo ER et al. Definition of phenotypic characteristics of childhood onset inflammatory bowel disease. *Gastroenterology* 2008 ;135:11144-22

[7]   Vernier-Massouille G, Balde M, Salleron J, et al. Natural history of pediatric Crohn's disease: a population-based cohort study. *Gastroenterology* 2008; 135:1106-1113.

[8]   Benchimol EI, Guttmann A, Griffiths AM, et al. Increasing incidence of pediatric inflammatory bowel disease in Ontario, Canada: evidence from health administrative data. *Gut* 2009; 58:1490-1497.

[9]   Phavichitr N, Cameron DJ, Catto-Smith AG. Increasing incidence of Crohn's disease in Victorian children. *J. Gastroenterol. Hepatol.* 2003; 18: 329–32.

[10]   Gearry RB, Richardson A, Frampton CM, Collett JA, Burt MJ, Chapman BA, Barclay ML. High incidence of Crohn's disease in Canterbury, New Zealand: results of an epidemiologic study. *Inflamm. Bowel Dis.* 2006; 12: 936-943.

[11] Ahuja V, Tandon RK. Inflammatory bowel disease in the Asia–Pacific area: A comparison with developed countries and regional differences. *J. Dig. Dis.* 2010; 11; 134–147.

[12] Rogers BMG, Clark LM, Kirsner JB. The epidemiologic and demographic characteristics of inflammatory bowel disease: an analysis of a computerized file of 1400 patients. *J. Chronic. Dis.* 1971; 24:743-773.

[13] Day AS, Whitten KE, Sidler M, Lemberg DA. Review article: Nutritional therapy in Paediatric Crohn's disease. *Aliment. Pharmacol. Ther*, 2008;27: 293-307.

[14] Griffiths AM. Specificities of inflammatory bowel disease in childhood. *Best Pract. Res. Clin. Gastroenterol.* 2004;18:509-23.

[15] Walters TD, Griffiths AM. Mechanisms of growth impairment in pediatric Crohn's disease. *Nat. Rev. Gastroenterol. Hepatol.* 2009; 6: 513–523.

[16] Nicholas DB, Otley A, Smith C, Avolio J, Munk M, Griffiths AM. Challenges and strategies of children and adolescents with inflammatory bowel disease: a qualitative examination. *Health Qual. Life Outcomes.* 2007 May 25;5:28.

[17] Otley A, Smith C, Nicholas D, Munk M, Avolio J, Sherman PM, Griffiths AM. The IMPACT questionnaire: a valid measure of health-related quality of life in pediatric inflammatory bowel disease. *J. Pediatr. Gastroenterol. Nutr.* 2002;35:557-63.

[18] Hilsden RJ, Verhoef MJ, Rasmussen H, Porcino A, DeBruyn JC. Use of complementary and alternative medicine by patients with inflammatory bowel disease. *Inflamm. Bowel Dis.* 2011;17:655-62.

[19] Hilsden RJ, Scott CM, Verhoef MJ. Complementary medicine use in patients with inflammatory bowel disease. *Am. J. Gastroenterol.* 1998; 93: 697-701.

[20] Hilsden RJ, Meddings JB, Verhoef MJ. Complementary and alternative medicine use by patients with inflammatory bowel disease: an internet survey. *Can. J. Gastroenterol.* 1999; 13: 327-32.

[21] Verhoef MJ, Scott CM, Hilsden RJ. A multimethod research study on the use of complementary and alternative therapies among patients with inflammatory bowel disease. *Altern. Ther. Health Meth.* 1998; 4: 68-71.

[22] Rawsthorne P, Shanahan F, Cronin NC, Anton PA, Löfberg R, Bohman L, Bernstein CN. An international survey of the use and attitudes regarding alternative medicine by patients with inflammatory bowel disease. *Am. J. Gastroenterol.* 1999;94:1298-303.

[23] Langmead L, Chitnis M, Rampton DS. Use of complementary therapies by patients with IBD may indicate psychological distress. *Inflam. Bowel Dis.* 2002; 8: 174-9.

[24] Limdi JK, Butcher RO. Complementary and alternative medicine use in Inflammatory Bowel Disease. *Inflamm. Bowel Dis.* 2011; 17: E86-88.

[25] Day AS. Use of complementary and alternative therapies by children attending gastroenterology outpatient clinics. *J. Paediatr. Child Health*, 2002;38:343-6.

[26] Wadhera V, Lemberg DA, Leach ST, Day AS. Complementary and Alternative Medicine in Children attending Gastroenterology Clinics: Usage Patterns and Reasons for Use. *J. Paediatr. Child Health.* 2011; 47: 904-910.

[27] Day AS, Whitten KE, Bohane TD. Use of complementary and alternative medicines by children and adolescents with Inflammatory Bowel Disease. *J. Paediatr. Child Health*, 2004;40: 681-4.

[28] Otley AR, Verhoef MJ, Best A et al. Prevalence and determinants of use of complementary and alternative medicine in a Canadian pediatric inflammatory bwel disease (IBD) population. *Gastroenterology*. 2011; 120: A213.

[29] Heuschkel R, Afzal N, Wuerth A, Zurakowski D, Leichtner A, Kemper K, Tolia V, Bousvaros A. Complementary medicine use in children and young adults with inflammatory bowel disease. *Am. J. Gastroenterol.* 2002; 97: 382-8.

[30] Markowitz JE, Mamula P, delRosario JF, Baldassano RN, Lewis JD, Jawad AF, Culton K, Strom BL. Patterns of complementary and alternative medicine use in a population of pediatric patients with inflammatory bowel disease. *Inflamm. Bowel. Dis.* 2004;10:599-605.

[31] Gerasimidis K, McGrogan P, Hassan K, Edwards CA. Dietary modifications, nutritional supplements and alternative medicine in paediatric patients with inflammatory bowel disease. *Aliment. Pharmacol. Ther.* 2008;27:155-65.

[32] Wong AP, Clark AL, Garnett EA, Acree M, Cohen SA, Ferry GD, Heyman MB. Use of complementary medicine in pediatric patients with inflammatory bowel disease: results from a multicenter survey. *J. Pediatr. Gastroenterol. Nutr.* 2009;48:55-60.

[33] Cotton S, Humenay Roberts Y, Tsevat J, Britto MT, Succop P, McGrady ME, Yi MS. Mind-body complementary alternative medicine use and quality of life in adolescents with inflammatory bowel disease. *Inflamm. Bowel. Dis.* 2010;16:501-6.

[34] Gilmour J, Harrison C, Asadi L, Cohen MH, Vohra S. Treating teens: considerations when adolescents want to use complementary and alternative medicine. *Pediatrics* 2011; 128 (Supp 4): S161-6.

[35] Evans A, Duncan B, McHugh P, Shaw J, Wilson C. Inpatients' use, understanding, and attitudes towards traditional, complementary and alternative therapies at a provincial New Zealand hospital. *NZ Med. J.* 121:21-34.

In: Alternative Medicine
Editors: Kenneth R. Carter and George E. Murphy

ISBN 978-1-62257-106-2
©2012 Nova Science Publishers, Inc.

Chapter 6

COMPLEMENTARY AND ALTERNATIVE MEDICINE APPROACHES IN THE TREATMENT OF CANCER

Sanjiv K. Duggal[1], Amritpal S. Saroya[*2] and Jaswinder S. Chauhan[3]*

[1]School of Applied Medical Sciences, Department of Pharmaceutical Sciences, Lovely Professional University, Phagwara, India
[2]School of Ayurveda, Department of Medicinal Plant Sciences, Sri Dhanwantry Ayurvedic College, Chandigarh, India
[3]Department of Pharmacology, Sri Guru Ram Das Institute of Medical Education and Research, Amritsar, India

ABSTRACT

"Complementary" and "Alternative" are terms used to describe a number of products, practices, and systems that are not part of mainstream (conventional, standard, or Western) medicine. They can include methods like herbs and dietary supplements, body movement, spiritual approaches, pills, extracts, and creams and ointments. Some are done by a person with extensive formal education and training (art therapy), while others may be recommended by the person who is selling the product in a store or on the Internet (colon therapy) or needles acupuncture) to no-touch "energy work" (reiki). Some are time-consuming or expensive (rigid diets or treatments in another country); others are fairly cheap and easy to use (vitamins or homeopathy). Some can be done at home on your own (meditation) and others require another person to give them (massage). Some almost never cause harm, while others can be dangerous and cause deaths.

Keywords: Cancer, CAM, chemoprevention, phytochemicals, phytopharmaceuticals, herbals

---

* Address for correspondence: Dr Amritpal Singh, 2101, Ph-7, Mohali-160062. Distt: Mohali (SAS Nagar). Mobile 9855203483. Email: amritpal2101@yahoo.com.

INTRODUCTION

Alternative medicine is used instead of standard medical treatment, often with serious consequences for the patient [1] Complementary medicine is used long with minstream medical care. Some complementary methods can also cause harm, but if carefully chosen and properly used, they might improve the quality of life [2]. According to a comprehensive survey on American's use of CAM, 36 per cent of U.S. adults are using some forms of CAM [3]. Survey found that rates of CAM use are especially high among pateints with serious illnesses such as cancer.

When megavitamin therapy and prayer for health reasons are included in the definition of CAM, that per centage rises to 62 per cent. The 69 per cent of 453 cancer patients had used at least one CAM therapy as part of their cancer treatment. 88 percent of 102 people with cancer had used one of he CAM therapies.

Of those 93 percent had used supplements, 53 percent had used non supplement forms of CAM and 47 percent has used both [4]

COMPLEMENTARY AND ALTERNATIVE METHODS FOR CANCER MANAGEMENT [5]

People with cancer can consider CAM for a number of reasons:

1. To releive the side effects of main stream cancer treatment.
2. To find a less unpleasent approach that has few or no side effects.
3. To take an active role in improving their own health and wellness.

Some complementary therapies may help to relieve certain symptoms of cancer, releive side effects of cancer therapy, or improve a patient's sense of well being. The American Cancer Society urges patients who are thinking about the use of any alternative or complementary therapy to discuss this with their health care team. Some alternative therapies have dangerous or even life-threatening side effects. With others, the main danger that the patient may lose to benefit from standard therapy [5]. Complementary approaches that are used with cancer treatment include Aromatherapy, biofeedback, botanical or herbal medicines, cartilage therapy, labyrinth walking, music therapy, Garson therapy, Essiac herbal formula, and nutritional supplements. Among several CAM anticancer approaches, botanical or herbal medicines, are widley used. Some evidence has accumulated for botanical or herbal medicines for their role in cancer treatment. Role of majoirty of the CAM approaches, in cancer treatment is not scientifically validated [6].

1. Essiac Herbal Formula [7, 8]

The formula originated among the Ojibwe people of North Amercia, one of whom gave it to a white woman about the turn of the last century. She in turn gave it to a highly qualified and experienced nurse in an Ontario hospital in 1992.

Table 1.

S.no	Medicinal Plant	Part used	Phytochemistry
1.	*Arctium lappa* L. (Asteraceae)	Root	Bitter glycoside: lappatin, sesquiterpene lactone: arctopicrin, fukinone, lignans: arctin, arctigenin, mateiresionol, arctiol, lappol, sterol:taraxasterol
2.	*Rheum officinale* L.(Polygonaceae)	Roots	Antharquinone derivatives: chrysophanic acid, emodin, rhein, calcium oxalate, oxalic acid, and resinous substance
3.	*Rumex acetosella* L.(Chenopodiaceae)	Roots	Antharquinone derivatives: lapathin and lapathin, calcium oxalate, oxalic acid, and resinous substance
4.	*Ulmus fulma* L. (Ulmaceae)		Tannins

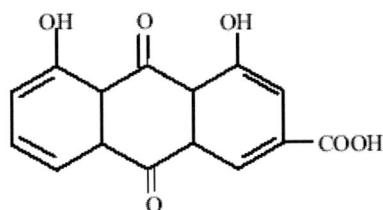
Rhein

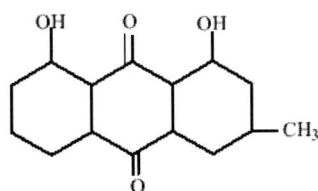
chrysophanol

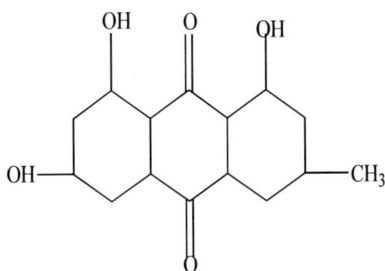
emodin

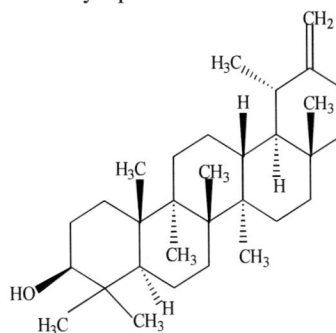
taraxasterol

Figure 1. Major phytochemicals of Essiac herbal formula.

The formula has been reported to be effective immunomodulator. Essiac does three things: it cleans the blood, cleans the liver and oxygentaes the cells. As result of taking it, a sick feels person feels more energetic and euphoric. Ingredients of Essiac herbal formula are as follows:

- Burdock, root (*Arctium lappa*)
- Sheep sorrel, leaf (*Rumex acetosella*)
- Slippery Elm, powder (*Ulmus fulma*)
- Turkey Rhubarb, root powder(*Rheum officinale*)
- Phytochemical profile of Essiac herbal formula

2. CARTILAGE

Cartilage is a type of tough, flexible connective tissue that forms parts of the skeleton in many animals. Cartilage contains cells called chondrocytes, which are surrounded by collagen and proteoglycans, which are made of protein and carbohydrate. Three theories have been proposed to explain how cartilage acts against cancer:

- As cartilage is broken down by the body, it releases products that kill cancer cells.
- Cartilage increases the action of the body's immnune system to kill cancer cells.
- Cartilage makes substances that block tumour angiogenesis (the growth of new blood vessels that feed a tumour and help it grow.

Based on laboratory and animals tuies, the third theory is most likely. Cartilage does not contain blood vessels, so cancer can not easily grow in it. It is suggested that a cancer treatment using cartilage may keep blood vessels from forming in a tumour, causing the tumour to stop growing or shrink.

In animal studies, cartilage products have been given by mouth; injected into a vein or the abdomen; applied to the skin; or placed in slow-release plastic pellets that were surgically implanted. In studies with people; cartilage products have been given by mouth; applied to skin; injected under the skin;or given by enema. The dose and length of time the cartilage treatment was given was different for each study, in part because of different types of products were used.

3. GERSON THERAPY [9]

Gerson therapy has been used by some people to treat has been to treat cancer and other diseases. It is based on the role of minerals, enzymes, and other dietary factors. There are 3 key parts to the therapy:

- *Diet*: Organic fruits, vegetables, and whole grains to give the body plenty of vitamins, minerals, enzymes, and other nutrients. The fruits and vegetables are low in sodium and high in pottasium.
- *Suppelemtation*: The addition of certain substances to the diet to help correct cell metabolism (the chemical changes that take place in a cell to make energy and basic materials needed for the body's life processes).
- *Detoxification*: Treatments, including enemas, to remove toxic substances from the body.

The Gerson therapy is based on the idea that cancer develops when there are changes in cell metabolism because of the build up of toxic substances in the body. According to Gerson, the disease process makes more toxins and the liver becomes overworked. Accordiong to Dr. Gerson, people with cancer also have too much solium and too little pottasium in the cells in their bodies, which causes tissue damage and weakend organs.

The goal of Gerson's therapy is to restore the body to health by repairing the liver and returning the metabolism to its normal state. It cane be done by removing toxins form the body and building up the immune system with diet and supplements.

The enemas are said to widen the the bile ducts of the heaptobiliary apparatus so that toxins can be released. The liver is furhter overworked as the treatment regimen breaks down the cancer cells abd rids the body of toxins. Pancreatic enzymes are given to decrease the demands on the weakened liver and pancreas to make enzymes for digestion.

4. SPECIFIC BOTANICALS

Mistletoe Extract [10]

Research study is being conducted to find out whether an extract of European mistletoe plant (*Viscum album* L.), along with with a chemotherapy drug called gemcitabine, can help treat people with certain cancers.

5. DIETARY PHYTOCHEMICALS

Recently, numerous reviews of plant derived chemopreventive compounds have identified their role in treatment of cancer. Thes chemopreventive compounds, precisely knon as phytopharaceuticals, are dietary ingredients, which being food derived, are considered pharmacologically safe [11] Some of the common chemopreventive dietary compounds derived from dietary ingredients are depicted in figure 114. Chemopreventive plant compounds affect all phases of the cancer process, i.e., tumor intiation, promotion and progression. Botanical medicines are complex natural mixtues of pharmacological musltitaskers, simulataneously exerting influence on different levels and via different mechanisms. By contrast, pharmaceutical drugs are classically single synthetic compounds, ideallyu intefering or disrupting specific mechanism [12].

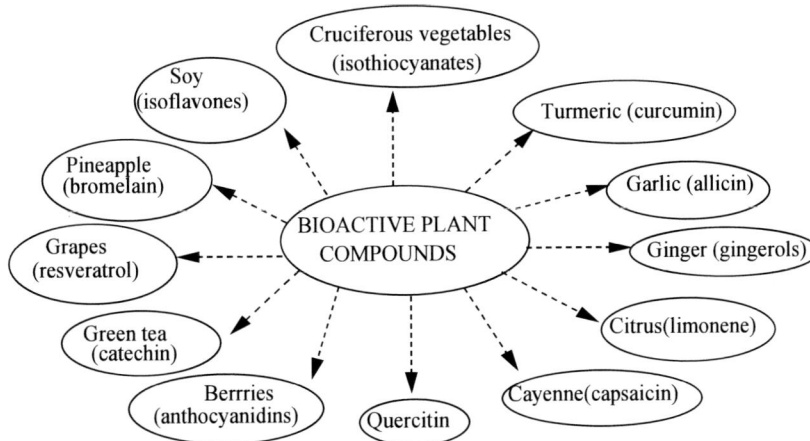

Figure 2. Common chemopreventive dietary compounds.

β-sitosterol

It is phytosterol. Epidemiological and experimental studies have suugested a protective role of β-sitosterol in the development of some types of cancer such as breast, colon and prostate.

In vivo studies have shown that β-sitosterol inhibited proliferation and induce apoptosis in colon and breast cancers. The studies clearly show that β-sitosterol kills breast cancer cells ad is not toxic to normal cell.

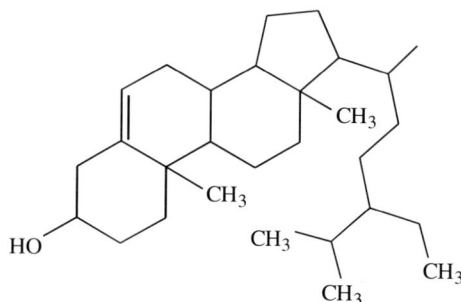

Figure 3. Structure of β-sitosterol.

Clinical srudies linking β-sitosterol and breast cancer are still missing but some scientists suggest that it may improve the efficiency of tamoxifrn, a drug of the used to treat breast cancer [13].

Curcumin

Dietary administration of this compound at a level of 2% to mice reduced the incidence of experimentally-induced colonic hyperplasia, indicating that the antioxidant effects are active in vivo. Curcumin inhibits cancer at initiation, promotion and progression stages of development.

Research has demonstrated that curcumin blocks the activity of a hormone having link with development of colorectal cancer. Other studies have demonstrated that curcumin inhibits melanoma cell growth and destroys cancer cells. In addition, animal research reported that curcumin prevented spread of breast cancer cells to lungs [5,16].

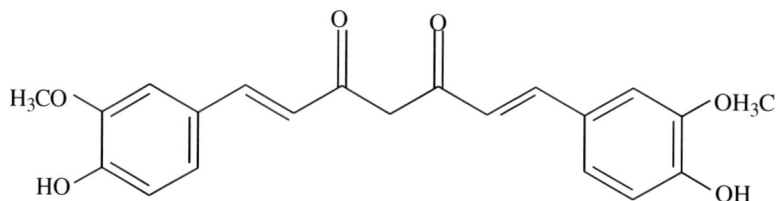

Figure 4. Structure of curcumin.

(-)-Epigallocatechin Gallate

(-)-Epigallocatechin gallate has an astringent effect and may inhibit cell membrane phosphorylation. The researchers do not know whether the polyphenols inhibit the initiation or the promotion of tumours. Tea also contains caffeine at a significant level (about 5%) and this has been shown to have a small tumour inhibiting effect. The proof is not confirmed, but the paper recommends the relaxing cup of tea anyway [14].

In this study the effects of green tea and its major components, (-)-epigallocatechin gallate and caffeine, on the tobacco-specific nitrosamine 4-(methylnitrosamino)-1-(3-pyridyl)-1-butanone (NNK)-induced lung tumorigenesis in A/J mice was examined. Inhibition by green tea and (-)-Epigallocatechin gallate in NNK-induced lung tumorigenesis is due at least partly to their antioxidant properties [15].

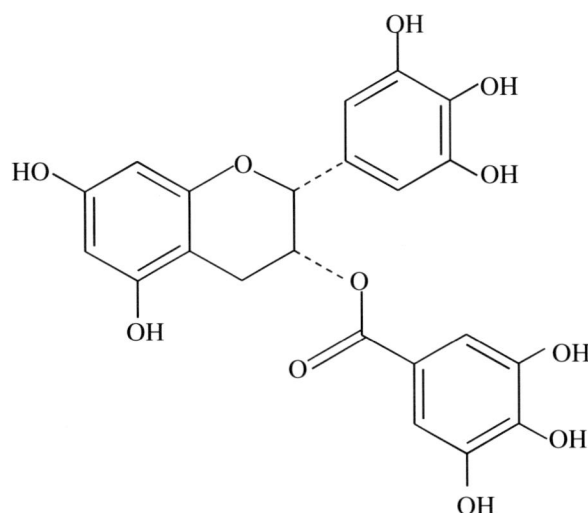

Figure 5. Structure of (-)-Epigallocatechin gallate.

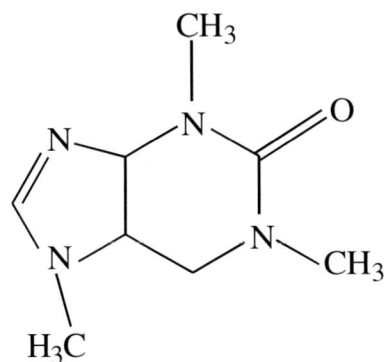

Figure 6. Structure of caffeine.

Resveratrol

It is a type of polyphenol called a phytoalexin, a class of compounds produced as part of a plant's defense systyem against disease. Resveratrol has been shown to reduce tumour incidence in animals by affecting one or more stages of cancer development. It has been shown to inhibit growth of many types of cancer cells in culture. Evidence also exists that it can reduce inflammation. It also reduces activation of NF κ B, a protein produced by the body's immune system when it is under attack. This protein affects cancer cell growth and metastasis [5, 16].

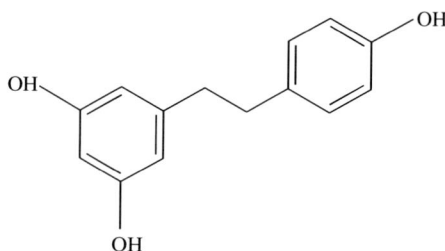

Figure 7. Structure of resveratrol.

Phytic Acid

Phytic acid's chelating effect may serve to prevent, inhibit, or even cure some cancers by depriving those cells of minerals, especially iron they need to reproduce. The deprivation of essential minerals like iron would, much like other broad treatments for cancer , also have negative effects on ono-cancerous cells [5, 16]

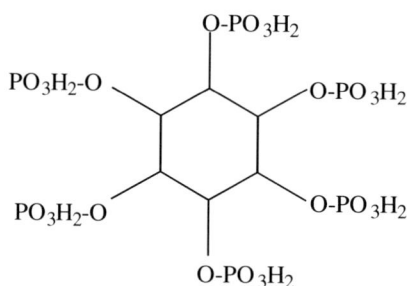

Figure 8. Structure of phytic acid.

Punicalagin

A recent animal study reported that ellagitannins present in fruit of pomegranate have possible protective role in prostate cancer. The researchers found that ellagitannins accumulate in the prostate and it may be mode of cancer prevention action. Punicalagin was suggested as possible anticancer agent [16]

S-allyl Cysteine

The key ingredient in garlic is S-allyl cysteine, which has been proven to protect against oxidation, free radicals, pollution, cancer and cardiovascular diseases.

It was found that S-allyl cysteine derived from Aged Garlic Extract inhibited the proliferation of nine human melanoma cell lines and one murine melanoma cell line in a dose dependent manner. S-allyl cysteine inhibited cellular growth and proliferation and modulated major cell differentiation marker of melanoma [17].

Phytochemicals of *Persea Americana* Mill (Avocado)

Recent studies reported that phytochemicals found in the fruit can prevent the onset of cancer and kill some cancer cells. Phytochemicals extracted from the fruit strike the multiple signaling pathways and prevent cancer by inducing diseases cell death.

The phytochemicals has no action on healthy cells. The fruit contains proteins (25%) vitamin C, vitamin E, unsaturated fatty acids and sesquiterpenes. The fruit is zero sodium [18]

CONCLUSION

Complementary and alternative therapies help to relieve certain symptoms of cancer, relieve side effects of cancer therapy, or improve a patient's sense of well being.

Side effects and ecomoncis of conebtional anticancer drugs have inspired the scientists to study plant or natural product derived or CAM therpies used in cancer, for potential and cost-effecive cures. Results obtained from studies with dietary phytochemcials are noteworthy and need further attention.

REFERENCES

[1]   World Health Organisation. *The promotion and development of traditional medicine*. Geneva: World Health Organization, 1978. (Technical reports series no. 622).

[2]   Wasik J. *The truth about herbal supplements*. Consumer's Digest. July/August 1999:75-79.

[3]   Flynn R, Roest M. *Your guide to standardized herbal products*. Prescott, AZ: One World Press, 1995.

[4]   Aggarwal BB, Takada Y, Oommen OV. From chemoprevention to chemo-therapy: common targets and common goals. *Expert Opinion.on Investigational. Drug.* 2004,13, 1327-1338.

[5]   Bagchi D, Preuss H. *Phytopharmaceuticals in Cancer Chemoprevention*. Boca Raton:CRC Press; 2005.

[6]   Weiner, M.A. and J.A. Weiner. *Herbs That Heal*. Quantum Books, Mill Valley, California.1994.

[7]   Hoad J. *Healing with Herbs*. Jaico Publishing House, New Dehli, 1997, pp:84-86.

[8]   Bell E A, Charlwood BV. *Secondary plant products* (Encyclop. Plant Physiology, Vol. Berlin-Heidelberg-New York: Springer Verlag, 1980.

[9]   Readers Digest : "The healing power of vitamins, minerals and herbs publishers by Readers digest Australia. Pvt. Ltd. Reprinted. 2001-02.

[10]   Bagchi D, Preuss H. *Phytopharmaceuticals in Cancer Chemoprevention.* Boca Raton:CRC Press; 2005. Bagchi D, Preuss H. *Phytopharmaceuticals in Cancer Chemoprevention.* Boca Raton:CRC Press; 2005.

[11]   Anonyms. The role of phytochemicals in optimal Health. *Journal of the National Academy for Child Development,* 1997;2.

[12]   Award AB, Barta SL, Fink CS, Bradford PG. β-sitosterol enhances tamoxifen effectiveness on breast cancer cells by affedting ceramide metabolism. *Journal of Molecular Nutrition and Food Research* 2008; 12:12-19.

[13]   Zhao BL, Li XJ, He RG, Cheng SJ, Xin WJ. Scavenging effect of extracts of green tea and natural antioxidants on active oxygen radicals. *Cellular Biophysics* 1989; 14(2):175-85.

[14]   Xu Y Ho CT Amin SG Han C Chung FL: Inhibition of tobacco-specific nitrosamine-induced lung tumorigenesis in A/J mice by green tea and its major polyphenol as antioxidants. *Cancer Research* 1992;52:3875-9.

[15]   Kuo P-Lin, Hsu Ya-Ling, Lin C. The Chemopreventive effects of natural products against human cancer cells. *International Journal of Applied Science and Engineering* 2005;3:203-214.

[16]   Takeyama H. et al. Growth Inhibition and Modulation of Cell Markers of Melanoma by S-allyl cysteine. *Oncology* 1993; 50:63-69.

[17]   Ding H. et al. *Chemo preventive characteristics of avocado fruit.* Seminars in Cancer Biology, 2007.

In: Alternative Medicine
Editors: Kenneth R. Carter and George E. Murphy

ISBN 978-1-62257-106-2
©2012 Nova Science Publishers, Inc.

Chapter 7

USE OF COMPLEMENTARY AND ALTERNATIVE MEDICINE FOR TREATMENT OF EPILEPSY

*Reyna M. Durón[1] and Kenton R. Holden[2]**

[1]Centro Médico Lucas, Tegucigalpa, Honduras, Central America,
Professional Advisory Board, Epilepsy Foundation of Greater Los Angeles, US
[2]Departments of Neurosciences (Neurology) and Pediatrics,
Medical University of South Carolina (MUSC), Charleston, South Carolina, US,
and Greenwood Genetic Center (GGC), Greenwood, South Carolina, US

ABSTRACT

Throughout the world, many people use complementary and alternative medicine (CAM) to treat epilepsy. One common CAM used is herbal medicine.

Although many plant ingredients are used in modern medications and some appear to have anticonvulsant properties, there are no evidence-based clinical studies that any control epileptic seizures. Difficulties with plant studies arise because concentrations of active principles can vary according to growing conditions. Some are also known to act on the cytochrome p450 system to alter plasma anti-epileptic drug (AED) levels, possibly detrimentally. Literature on other CAMs used in epilepsy is readily available.

Acupuncture studies in animals reveal antiepileptic effects and are likely secondary to altering neurotransmission. Prayer, music, and relaxation techniques are also frequently used CAMs. Vitamins and minerals can help prevent some secondary effects of AEDs. Ketogenic and Atkins diets have been found to be useful evidence-based CAM treatments in refractory epilepsies of children and adults. Surveys from Asia, Europe, and the United States have shown that 35 to 72% of patients with severe or refractory neurological disorders use CAM, although many do not report it to their physicians.

* Correspondence: Kenton R. Holden, M.D., Professor, Departments of Neurosciences (Neurology) and Pediatrics, Medical University of South Carolina (MUSC), Charleston, SC, USA and Senior Clinical Research Neurologist, Greenwood Genetic Center (GGC), Greenwood, SC, USA. E-mail: holdenk@musc.edu or kholden@ggc.org.

This percentage is similar for patients with epilepsy, who commonly switch to CAM or combine CAM with prescribed medications. The chance that CAM will be used for an illness appears related to experience with CAM use in the past and a belief in the safety of CAM use. Patients with advanced education degrees beyond upper school appear to have a higher prevalence of CAM use.

Commonly patients think that CAMs are safer, more "natural", and lack secondary adverse effects. However, most CAM use is likely precipitated by dissatisfaction with failed evidence-based medical treatments, lack of access to or unavailability of AEDs, inadequate education about epilepsy, insufficient resources, and cultural beliefs. Cultures which believe in diseases caused by "the supernatural" use traditional medicine/CAM as initial therapy rather than of modern medical therapies.

CAM use to treat epilepsy has five possible outcomes to the patient. First, their effect is neutral or not harmful and/or they do not interact with an AED or other modern epilepsy treatments. Second, their effect is detrimental to the patient because of direct effects or undesired interactions. Third, they are not effective as an AED, but they do promote general health. Fourth, their effect is unknown, and, therefore, most likely risky. Fifth, they are effective as an AED. CAM use in epilepsy patients often is related to non-adherence to evidence-based AED treatment. Because of the wide range of CAM effects, patients and medical providers need to discuss openly the use of CAM in the treatment of epilepsy. A comprehensive epilepsy education program is needed initially to change non-adherent behaviors and to close the treatment gap for epilepsy.

This must go hand-in-hand with improved access to resources and treatment. At the same time, clinical translational research needs to be promoted to determine newer specific and adjuvant therapies for epilepsy, some of which may prove to be CAMs currently in use.

INTRODUCTION

Many people over the world use complementary and alternative medicine (CAM) to treat acute and chronic illnesses. Since neurological diseases are common (epilepsy, stroke, head trauma, developmental, etc.) and many times do not respond to conventional therapy, CAMs are commonly used. Epilepsy is no exception. Surveys from Asia, Europe, and the United States have shown that 35 to 72% of patients with severe or refractory neurological disorders use CAM, although many do not report it to their physicians. [Barnes et al, 2004] This percentage is similar for patients with epilepsy, who commonly switch to CAM or combine CAM with prescribed medications. [Durón et al, 2009] Traditions, beliefs, and psychosocial factors contribute to treatment practices of epilepsy. These factors appear to differ between developed and developing nations. Even when people migrate from underdeveloped to developed countries, they tend to retain cultural beliefs and treatment practices about epilepsy similar to those in their home countries. Individuals who believe in non-scientific causes of epilepsy tend to initially use complementary and alternative medical therapies. Sometimes, this can lead to risks to health and to diminished quality of life.

Epilepsy is a common worldwide health problem; however the etiological causes can differ between developed and developing nations. Recent reports conclude that undeveloped regions, such as parts of Latin America, Asia, and Africa, have higher epilepsy prevalence rates as a result of "preventable" epilepsies.[Medina et al, 2005; Bergen, 1998]

Studies in countries like Honduras, Central America also reflect the impact of patient and community perceptions about epilepsy. When 2,221 persons from the Honduran Miskito tribe were evaluated during a population-based epilepsy prevalence study and compared to hospital and governmental clinic records, it was found that the epilepsy prevalence was much lower than expected [Varela et al, 2002]. It was also observed that there was a strong tendency to explain epilepsy using magical and religious terms and to also use traditional treatments.

This study serves as an example of how carefully data needs to be obtained and results reported in epidemiological studies, particularly in certain populations. The social interaction of epilepsy patients with their community and the stigma associated with epilepsy in their community may play a major role in the outcomes of any specific reports on the use of modern medications or CAMs for epilepsy.

Additional anthropological studies on epilepsy in different parts of the world have reported that people with epilepsy are frequently believed to be unable to carry on a normal profession or to be independent in everyday tasks [Devinski and Cramer, 1993; Dodrill, 1993].

Psychosocial problems stemming from the epilepsies vary among countries and ethnic groups [Lai and Lai, 1991; Pal et al, 2008; Collins, 1994; Elferink, 1999; Durón et al, 2001]. Earlier literature from African countries, for example, reported that epilepsy has frequently been treated as an abomination, and there is evidence that in many areas it continues to be abhorred and highly stigmatized [Jilek-Aall et al, 1997; Osuntokun, 1977]. Belief remains strong in many regions of the world that only traditional healers are capable of divining the causes and treating the condition. Literature indicates that in rural areas, relatives and family members sometimes accept seizure disorders as a misfortune and do not accept modern medical attention.

Use of herbs and non-pharmacological CAMs have been reported by patients everywhere. Since CAM use is common in epilepsy patients, doctors and other allied health personnel should make an effort to learn about it in order to instruct patients, and, if applicable, to rationally use those measures that could be helpful for well being and stress reduction, if not for seizure control.

Some complementary treatments are currently helpful in preventing chronic AED adverse effects such as anemia, osteopenia, osteoporosis, and teratogenesis.

REASONS FOR CAM USE IN EPILEPSY

In developed countries, the search for alternative treatments is initiated primarily due to lack of seizure control from modern AEDs. In addition, CAM use is increased because the most commonly used AEDs can have adverse effects such as allergic reactions, gingival hyperplasia, gastrointestinal disturbances, osteopenia or osteoporosis, bone marrow toxicity, liver toxicity, nephrotoxicity, neurological symptoms (ataxia, dizziness, diplopia, somn-olence), cognitive, mood, and behavioral disturbances, endocrine dysfunction, and terato-genicity. Other non-pharmacological evidence-based treatments of epilepsy such as the Ketogenic diet, vagal nerve stimulator, and epilepsy surgery have their own limitations and complications, and many in the world cannot access these evidence-based antiepileptic therapies.

**Table 1. Epilepsy patient and non-patient beliefs about the cause
of epilepsy in two cohorts from 3 communities in the rural
Department of Olancho, Honduras**

Responses	Epilepsy patients n=90	Non-patients n=190
Do not know	38	43
Parasites "bad worm" and/or neurocysticercosis	21	13
Heredity	7	19
Cerebral fatigue	4	3
Problems in blood	0	18
Head trauma	4	5
Weakness	2	6
Sorcery, witchcraft, demons, spirits	2	26
Nervousness, anxiety	0	14
Not eating, bad nutrition	2	4
Careless practices*	3	32
Contact with dead bodies	0	4
Drugs, alcohol	0	4
Lack of sexual activity	0	10
Other**	15	59

* Like taking a bath immediately after physical activity.

** Digestive problems, congenital defects, exposure to cold wind, use of forceps during birth, fever, unexpected events/news, lack of menses, problems with husband or family problems, taking a bath during menses, malaria, temperature changes.

Cultures which believe in diseases caused by "the supernatural" inherently feel the need for traditional medicine/CAM rather than modern medicine. Although probably more likely used in developing countries, the chance that CAM will be used for an illness appears related to the patient's experience with CAM use in the past and a belief in the safety of CAM use. It is of interest that in developed countries, patients with advanced education degrees appear to have a higher prevalence of CAM use. Commonly patients interpret that CAM options are safer because they are "natural". They consider CAMs to lack secondary adverse effects although very few controlled evidence-based studies support this premise. There are some patients who use herbal and dietary supplements for health promotion rather than to specifically treat their epilepsy. Other than that group, however, the "treatment gap" related to evidence-based epilepsy treatment primarily arises from the following factors: dissatisfaction with failed evidence-based medical treatments, lack of access or unavailability of AEDs, inadequate education about epilepsy, insufficient resources, and regional and cultural beliefs. These are also the factors which likely precipitate most CAM use. These reasons can be readily found both in developing and developed countries throughout the world.

There is a diversity of factors influencing CAM use for epilepsy and there is diversity in the specific CAM chosen. Epilepsy patients and normal community members from across the developing country of Honduras, including two tribal groups, were asked what they thought caused epilepsy [Durón et al, 2001, 2009; Varela et al, 2002]. Multiple responses from an individual were accepted.

Their responses, found in Table 1 and Table 2, indicate their beliefs about epilepsy. These beliefs may explain, in part, the stigma involved and may contribute to the treatment gap and CAM use found in these communities.

Table 2. Choice of complementary and alternative medicine (CAM) from a national survey of Honduran out-patients with epilepsy related to their community type (urban versus rural)

	Urban		Rural		Total	
	No.	%	No.	%	No.	%
Herbs	20	28.6	38	53.5	58	41.1
Potions	14	20.0	27	38.0	41	29.1
Amulets	1	1.4	1	1.4	2	1.4
Medicine man bath	2	2.9	6	8.5	8	5.7
Acupuncture	0	0.0	0	0.0	0	0.0
Massage with oils ("sobada")	1	1.4	4	5.6	5	3.5
Pray to saints	4	5.7	12	16.9	16	11.3
Pray to spirits	3	4.3	8	11.3	11	7.8
Pray to God	42	58.6	38	53.5	80	56.7
Special diet	3	4.3	5	7.0	8	5.7
Other	2	2.9	7	9.9	9	6.4

Table 3. Choice of first-aid (multiple responses from an individual were recorded) during an acute epileptic seizure obtained from Miskito tribesmen (n=49) without epilepsy from rural Honduras

	No.	%
Spray water on patient	22	45
Give Miskito medicine	20	41
Take patient to clinic	11	22
Spray aromatic substances	10	20
Tie or restrain the patient	4	8
"Lock" the patient	3	6
Put herbs on eyes (cilantro or garlic)	3	6
Blowing air	2	4
Give medicines or pills	2	4
Give intravenous liquids	2	4
Watch out for harás	2	4
Hold the patient	1	2
Make the patient calm	1	2
Massage hands with salt	1	2
Pray	1	2
Does not know what to do	3	6

**Table 4. Adherence history and CAM* use frequency for epilepsy
from a national (urban and rural) survey of out-patients with epilepsy
throughout all regions of Honduras**

	No.	%
Currently taking medicine	256	93.4
Had abandoned medicine sometime	121	44.2
Gets the medicine all the time	223	81.4
Use of CAM* sometime	141	51.5
Use of CAM* currently	86	31.4

*CAM = complementary and alternative medicine.

**Table 5. Reasons listed from a checklist for non-adherence to their antiepileptic drug(s)
from a national (urban and rural) survey of out-patients with epilepsy
throughout all regions of Honduras**

	No.	%
Drug not available at hospital	25	20.7
Drug not available at health center	25	20.7
No money to pay for drug	20	16.5
Thought drug didn't work	16	13.2
Forgot to take drug	16	13.2
Did not want to buy drug	15	12.4
Feared reaction to drug	14	11.6
Did not want to take drug	10	8.3
No transportation to get drug	9	7.4
No symptoms	8	6.6
Couldn't find a place selling drug	8	6.6
No time to get drug	7	5.8
"Other"[*]	4	3.4

[*]No prescription; drug expired.

CAM use is even part of first aid for acute epileptic seizures according to a tribe cohort of 49 non-epilepsy Miskito tribesmen from rural Honduras (Table 3). Additional national survey data taken from Honduran epilepsy out-patients show in Table 4 that CAM use from non-adherence to antiepileptic drugs (AEDs) relates not only to sociocultural aspects but to financial hardship and the treatment gap. Table 5 shows reasons for non-adherence to AED in Honduras [Durón et al, 2009]. Whether data was collected in rural or urban centers, the reasons for non-adherence to evidence-based AEDs, as well as the reasons for a high use of CAMs, is multifactorial and not easily solved by financial resources alone. Understanding why patients and their relatives chose CAM use as a substitute for epilepsy treatment will help develop educational strategies to overcome non-adherent issues.

CAMs and Evidence

Herbal Medicines

One of the most common CAMs is herbal medicine. Although many plants have contributed ingredients to modern medications, there is no strong consensus of clinical studies that support their use to control epileptic seizures. A recent Cochrane review analyzed 5 epilepsy herbal treatment trials for epilepsy. Although the methodology was not ideal a few studies showed results which seemed to exhibit some benefit by Far Eastern herbal remedies. Still, current evidence was insufficient to support its use to treat epilepsy [Li et al, 2009]. However, some appeared to have anticonvulsant properties in experimental models [Wong, 2010].

Animal studies reported from around the world have exhibited *in vitro* anticonvulsant effects of plants like *Capparis deciduas, Solanum nigrum, Croton zambesicus, Nylandtia spinosa L. Dumont, Ficus platyphylla, nutmeg oil of Myristica fragrans, Carissa edulis, Rosa damascene*, American skullcap (*Scutellaria lateriflora L.*), *Petiveria alliacea L., Acanthus montanus, Alchornea laxiflora, Hyptis spicigera, Microglossa pyrifolia, Piliostigma reticulatum, Voacanga Africana*, and others [Bum et al, 2009].

Other reports show anxiolytic and anticonvulsant effects on mice of flavonoids, linalool, and alpha-tocopherol that are present in the extract of leaves of *Cissus sicyoides L* [de Almeida et al, 2009] . Research has also suggested that the anticonvulsant properties shown by *L. alba* might be correlated to the presence of a complex of non-volatile substances (phenylpropanoids, flavonoids and/or inositols), and also to the volatile terpenoids (beta-myrcene, citral, limonene and carvone), which have been previously validated as anticonvulsants [Neto et al, 2009]. Animal models have shown the anticonvulsant properties of *Bacopa monnieri* extracts and *Ficus religios*, supporting that 5-HT(2C) receptors are novel targets for developing anti-convulsant drugs [Singh and Goeal, 2009].

The Q'eqchi' Maya health system in Central America and Mexico uses a large selection of plants to treat neurological disorders, including epilepsy and anxiety disorders. Canadian researchers have reported a study that evaluated ethanol extracts of 34 plants that were tested *in vitro* [Awad et al, 2009]. Ten plants showed greater than 50% GABA-T inhibition at 1mg/ml, while 23 showed greater than 50% binding to the GABA(A)-BZD receptor at 250 microg/ml. *Piperaceae, Adiantaceae* and *Acanthaceae* families were highly represented and active in both assays. This suggested a positive correlation between GABA-T inhibition and relative frequency of use for epilepsy [Awad et al, 2009]. Similar findings regarding potential antiseizure effects have been reported in a study on the effect of hydro-methanolic percolated extract of *Matricaria recutita L.* on seizures induced by picrotoxin in male mice [Grundman et al, 2008; Heidari et al, 2009]. Several other plants also appear to have anticonvulsant and antianxiety effects due to enhanced GABA effect. [Awad et al, 2009]

Resveratrol (Res) is a phytoalexin produced naturally by several plants that has been reported to offer neuroprotection, anti-inflammatory, and anti-cancer effects. A study reported that it showed an anti-epileptic effect against rat kainate-induced temporal lobe epilepsy (TLE). It showed protection of neurons against kainate-induced neuronal cell death in CA1 and CA3a regions and depressed mossy fiber sprouting, which are characteristic both in TLE patients and animal models. Western blot revealed that the expression level of kainate receptors (KARs) in the hippocampus was reduced in Res-administrated rats compared to that in the epileptic group.. These results suggest that plant phytoalexin is a potential anti-epilepsy agent with anti-epileptogenesis properties [Wu et al, 2009].

Even though promising results have been shown in pharmacologic and animal studies, difficulties which have been encountered in studies of using herbal medicines for patients with epilepsy include: 1) some herbs are rare or an endangered species, 2) herbs used today may not even correspond to the plants originally described in the old literature, 3) preparations may be from herbs that went through different breeding procedures over several centuries or had different environmental/growing conditions, 4) developing a therapeutic remedy from herbal origins is a complex process that includes standardization of the herbal extract, providing evidence of pharmacological activity, and providing evidence of safety, 5) knowing pharmacokinetic aspects of absorption, knowing the process of the biotrans-formation of the extract in the body, metabolism, and excretion, 6) the metabolism and pharmacokinetic behavior of active constituents may differ from species to species, and 7) countries define herbal medicines differently and have adopted various approaches to licensing, dispensing, manufacturing, and trading these products.

Some plant products have been shown to act on the cytochrome p450 system to alter plasma anti-epileptic drug (AED) levels in epilepsy patients and increase the risk of seizures through direct (pre-convulsant or altered AED metabolic properties) or indirect (contami-nation with heavy metals or other toxic substances) mechanisms.

Table 6 summarizes these and other effects of herbal compounds as reported in the current medical literature [Samuels et al, 2008; Tyai and Delanty, 2009; NLM, 2010a, 2010b]. In a recent reported US study of herb and dietary supplement use in patients with epilepsy, approximately one-third of patients used products that had the potential to increase seizures or interact with normal drug metabolism. [Kaiboriboon et al, 2009].

The effectiveness and safety of herbal medications for the treatment of epilepsy remains unanswered definitively, especially when used in combination with AEDs. These issues remain in need of much larger, higher quality randomized clinical trials than have been published to date.

At this point in time, the known adverse effects and central nervous system drug interactions with herbs should be studied by physicians and allied health personnel and discussed with patients (Table 6). Some specific plants have strong (grade A), good (grade B) or unclear (grade C) scientific evidence of their usefulness.

Individual consideration should be carefully evaluated when allowing herbs (chamomile, valerian, passiflora) to treat anxiety or insomnia in epilepsy patients, since they could have enhanced sedation effects. In addition, antidepressant drugs are commonly used in epilepsy patients, and their interactions with herbs also need be considered. It is not unusual for patients who use polypharmacy of any type to have unexpected or unexplained adverse side effects, whereas if with the same medications were used alone, the effects would be beneficial.

Table 6. A compendium of possible side effects and interactions of commonly used complementary and alternative medicine (CAM) with antiepileptic drugs as well as with other psychopharmacologic medications/compounds

Common name	Scientific name	Common secondary effects	Interactions
Animal or vegetable oils		None	Interference with intestinal absorption of drugs.
Chamomile	*Matricaria recutita, Chamomilla recutita*	Sedation can occur.	Sedation enhanced when combined with AEDs that cause drowsiness (benzodiazepines, barbiturates). May interfere with the cytochrome P450 liver enzyme system, serum levels of AEDs may be increased, with potential increased effects.
Eucalyptus oil	*E. Fructicetorum, Eucalyptus globulus* and other species	Gastrointestinal upset, dizziness, muscle weakness, constricted pupils, difficulty breathing, cough, cyanosis, delirium, or convulsions. Less commonly, drowsiness, hyperactivity, difficulty walking, slurred speech, and headache.	Increased drowsiness when taken with benzodiazepines, barbiturates, narcotics, some antidepressants, or alcohol. Interference with the cytochrome P450 enzyme system; serum levels of some drugs like barbiturates could be decreased.
Ephedra	*Ephedra sinica,* ma huang	Abdominal discomforts, anxiety, dizziness, headache, tremor, insomnia, dry mouth, delirium, fainting, irritability, euphoria, hallucinations, seizures, stroke, hypokalemia, hyperreflexia, weakness, muscle damage, depression, mania, suicidal ideas, Parkinson's disease-like symptoms, kidney stones, hypoglycemia, cardiac arrhythmia, high blood pressure, heart ischemia, myopathy, and cardiac arrest.	Severe cardiovascular and systemic reactions if combined with stimulants, MAOI antidepressants, alkaloids, anesthetic drugs, or antipsychotic drugs. Other antidepressants and medications for psychiatric disorders (phenothiazines, tricyclics, SSRIs) may reduce the effects of ephedra causing low blood pressure and tachycardia. Combination with caffeine may be fatal.
Echinacea	*Echinacea angustifolia DC, Echinacea pallida, Echinacea purpurea*	Few side effects reported. Complaints include stomach discomfort, sore throat, rash, drowsiness, headache, dizziness, liver dysfunction, thrombotic thrombocytopenic purpura, leukopenia, and muscle aches.	May affect liver metabolism of some drugs including an AED like valproate.
Evening primrose oil		Seizures could occur in individuals with previous seizure disorder, or in individuals receiving antipsychotics or anesthetics. Some report occasional headache, abdominal pain, nausea, and loose stools.	Increased risk of seizures when combined with chlorpromazine, thioridazine, trifluoperazine, fluphenazine, or general anesthesia. Anti-seizure medications may require adjustment because this herb increases risk of seizures. Possible additive effects may occur with anticoagulants, antidepressants, CNS stimulants, and drugs metabolized by the liver.
Ginkgo	*Ginkgo biloba L.*	Few and mild adverse effects like headache, nausea, intestinal complaints, bleeding, and rarely, hypoglycemia, and hypotension. Eating the seeds is potentially deadly, due to risk of tonic-clonic seizures and loss of consciousness.	Potential reduction of anti-seizure properties of sodium valproate or carbamazepine. This could be due to altered liver metabolism. Enhanced effects of MAOI drugs, SSRIs, anticoagulants, antiplatelet/aggregation drugs, non-steroidal anti-inflammatory drugs.

Table 6. (Continued)

Common name	Scientific name	Common secondary effects	Interactions
Ginseng	American ginseng, Asian ginseng, Panax ginseng and other	Long-term use may be associated with skin rash, diarrhea, sore throat, loss of appetite, excitability, blood hypertension, hypoglycemia, bleeding, anxiety, depression, or insomnia. Other side effects include headache, dizziness, chest pain, difficult menstruation, breast tenderness, vaginal bleeding after menopause (estrogen-like effects), heartburn, tachycardia, nausea, vomiting, or manic episodes in people with bipolar disorder.	Seizures have occurred after high consumption of energy drinks containing caffeine, guarana, and herbs, including ginseng. Headache, tremors, mania, or insomnia may occur if combined with MAOIs antidepressants. Potential effect on drug metabolism, by interference with the cytochrome P450 enzyme system, serum levels of certain drugs like AEDs could increase. Ginseng may interact with sedating drugs (like several AEDs).
Kava	*Piper methysticum* G. Forst	Liver toxicity including liver failure. Other serious side effects reported include: skin disorders, blood abnormalities, apathy, kidney damage, seizures, psychotic syndromes, pulmonary hypertension, high blood pressure, meningismus, and kidney toxicity. Mild side effects may include gastrointestinal upset or allergic rash. There are reports of abnormal muscle movements after short-term use, with rigidity, twisting, torticollis, and oculogyric crisis.	Potential increased risk of liver damage if taken with drugs that may affect the liver (such as the AED valproate). AEDs metabolized in kidneys should be used cautiously. There is potential increase in the effects of alcohol and drugs that cause sedation and interference with the cytochrome P450 system, which could increase serum levels of some AEDs.
Passiflora, Passion flower	*Passiflora incarnata L.*	Tachycardia, nausea, vomiting, drowsiness, sedation, mental slowing. Potential risk of bleeding and alteration of blood tests that measure blood clotting.	Some alkaloids with MAOI action present in some species of *Passiflora*, could enhance MAOI drugs. Increased sedation or low blood pressure could occur when combined with tricyclic antidepressants. There is interaction with sedative drugs (like benzodiazepines and barbiturates), also with drugs metabolized by the liver.
St. John's wort	*Hypericum perforatum L.*	Infrequent gastrointestinal upset, skin reactions, fatigue, sedation, anxiety, sexual dysfunction, photosensitivity, dizziness, headache, blood hypertension, and dry mouth. Some have reported psychiatric symptoms such as suicidal and homicidal thoughts.	Interference with the cytochrome P450 enzyme system, potential increase in serum levels of drugs like carbamazepine, cyclosporin, midazolam, nifedipine, simvastatin, theophylline, warfarin, or HIV drugs. Combination with antidepressants may lead to increased side effects, including serotonin syndrome and mania.
Valerian	*Valeriana officinalis L.* and other	Headache, excitability, stomach upset, uneasiness, dizziness, ataxia, hypothermia. Chronic use may cause insomnia. Slight transient reductions in concentration or complicated thinking may occur.	Drowsiness may be worsened when taken with sedating medications (benzodiazepines, barbiturates, and other), as a result of GABA enhancement. Potential liver toxicity could affect several drugs metabolism.

Key: SSRI = selective serotonin reuptake inhibitor; MAOI = monoamine oxidase inhibitor; AED = antiepileptic drug; CNS = central nervous system; GABA = gamma-aminobutyric acid; HIV = human immunodeficiency virus.

Samuels et al, 2008; Tyagi and Delanty , 2003; NLM 2010a, 2010b.

Acupuncture

Acupuncture is an ancient practice introduced by the Chinese culture. New or modified modalities include electroacupuncture, laser acupuncture, acupressure, and catgut implantation to acupoints. It has become an inexpensive and generally safe procedure. According to a recent review of complementary and alternative medicine use in the US population, an estimated 2.1 million people or 1.1% of the population sought acupuncture care during the past 12 months. Four percent of the US population have used acupuncture at some time in their lives [Barnes et al, 2004]

Acupuncture is based on beliefs regarding the regulation of five main elements (fire, earth, metal, water, and wood), as well as yin and yang, Qi, and blood and body fluids. It is thought that stimuli to some meridian points can bring internal homeostasis to the body systems. Some studies in animals and humans have shown that responses can occur both close to the site of application and at a distance, mediated mainly by sensory neurons to many structures within the central nervous system. There are several theories about the suspected inhibitory effect of acupuncture in seizures related to increasing the release of inhibitory neurotransmitters. Although animal studies using acupuncture reveal antiepileptic effects, suggesting that suppression of epileptic discharges is secondary to altering neurotransmission, a recent Cochrane review of 11 published studies concludes that acupuncture has not been proven to be safe or effective in treating people with epilepsy [Ceuk et al, 2009]. To date, the evidence in favor of acupuncture is more anecdotal than scientific. Randomized double-blinded studies are needed. With such widespread use of acupuncture at the present time, it should be a priority to adequately study whether or not there is a rational acupuncture protocol for specific ages and specific epilepsy types [Jindal et al, 1997].

Psychological-Behavioral

Biofeedback, prayer, yoga, music, and other similar therapies could be considered behavioral treatments for epilepsy. They are low-cost, noninvasive, ambulatory interventions that can be used simultaneously with standard treatments of epilepsy [Ramaratnam et al, 2001]. These techniques can enhance body and mind health, while at the same time possibly help decrease brain electrical activity which correlates with seizures. They can also be used in different cultural contexts. Biofeedback relaxation or imagery techniques have been found to be useful for anxiety, stress, headache pain, and hypertension which are common comorbidities in epilepsy patients. However, in recent Cochrane reviews of relaxation therapy, cognitive behavioral therapy, electroencephalographic or galvanic skin response biofeedback, as well as yoga as a treatment for control of epilepsy, used alone or in combination, no impact on seizure control was demonstrated. Although these interventions may reduce anxiety, improve social behavior, and improve compliance, further large well-designed high quality randomized clinical trails are needed to give these therapies reliable evidence to support them for the treatment of epilepsy [Yardi, 2001; Lundgren et al, 2008].

Vitamins and Other Dietary Supplements

Vitamins and minerals can help prevent some secondary effects of AEDs, eg, anemia, osteoporosis, and teratogenesis, and are necessary for good health. However, large doses of vitamins do not improve the symptoms of epilepsy and may even be harmful if given in megadoses. A balanced diet should supply most of the vitamins and minerals a person needs each day. People with epilepsy taking AEDs appear to have an increased need for folic acid, calcium, and vitamin D. Women who may become pregnant and pregnant women with and without epilepsy need sufficient folic acid to help prevent birth defects, especially those related to the brain and spinal cord.

The conclusion of a recent meta-analysis [AAN, 2009] was that the risk of spinal cord/brain anomalies in the offspring of women with epilepsy is possibly decreased by folic acid supplementation (two adequately sensitive Class III studies). Therefore, it is recommended that preconceptional folic acid supplementation or fortification in women with epilepsy be considered so as to reduce the risk of brain/spinal cord birth defects, especially meningomyelocele. Although the data are insufficient to show that it is effective in women with epilepsy, there is no evidence of the harm and no reason to suspect that it would not be effective in this group. There is no reason to modify the current folic acid supplementation or fortification recommendation that all women of childbearing potential, with or without epilepsy, receive supplementation or fortification with at least 0.4 mg of folic acid daily prior to conception and during pregnancy.

Melatonin, a natural hormone secreted by the brain's pineal gland, has been thought to reduce the incidence of epilepsy in children. Although there is no large meta-analysis to support the use of melatonin at this time for epilepsy therapy, further randomized control studies need to be done with this compound. Melatonin is of special interest since it plays a role in our normal sleep-awake cycle. Many epilepsy patients have additional seizures when they are sleep-deprived. Melatonin may offer in the future a unique opportunity for its use in a subgroup of epilepsy patients if evidence is forthcoming from future treatment trials to support its use.

Alternative Diets

Ketogenic and Atkins diets, as well as modifications of these diets, are useful evidence-based CAM therapies for use in refractory epilepsies of children and adults. The Ketogenic diet was initially used in 1921 as a way to cause diet-induced ketosis to mimic fasting, something known since biblical days as a treatment for epilepsy. Approximately 90% of the calories in the Ketogenic diet are derived from fat intake. Although the diet became less popular with the introduction of effective pharmacotherapy, it still remains an effective evidence-based therapy for seizures refractory to AEDs. The Ketogenic diet reduces seizure frequency by > 50% in 54% of children with intractable epilepsy [Vining et al, 2008; Freeman et al, 2009]. Although the diet is most effective in infants and young children, success can be found in all age groups. The anti-convulsant mechanism of action is still not known. However, a recent report on mice of the prevention by the Ketogenic diet of myopathic ultrastructural abnormalities from mitochondrial dysfunction appears to be important news in the quest to find an answer to the exact mechanism of action [Ahola-Erkkilä et al, 2010].

The modified Atkins diet [Kossoff et al, 2008] is high in fat and low in carbohydrates (low-carb) and has even been found to be useful for developing countries.

This modified diet resembles Dr. Atkins' low-carb diet designed for both weight loss and healthy living. The "Modified Atkins" diet for seizures can be viewed as a "lighter dose" of the Ketogenic diet. More highly studied in children, this less restrictive diet when compared to the Ketogenic diet reduces childhood seizure frequency by > 50% in 47% of children with intractable epilepsy. Adult studies are currently underway and preliminary reports are positive for its effectiveness for seizure control in this population too. Additional studies are also currently underway for other modified diets e.g., low-glycemic index, etc. to find a more tolerable diet that may be more or at least as effective as the Ketogenic diet.

Miscellaneous Therapies ("Other")

There are other CAMs reported by patients which will not be discussed in detail in this chapter. Although they commonly appear on "news" wires and on various "web-sites", therapies such as magnetotherapy, chiropractic, aromatherapy, homeopathy, desensitization and other condition strategies, focal cooling, etc. have had no rigorous scientific studies which conclude that any of them are beneficial in the control of epilepsy.

CAM USEAGE OUTCOMES

Health personnel and patients and/or their relatives need to remember the following about CAM usage outcomes. There are five possible results in the patient from using CAMs to treat epilepsy. *First*, their effect is neutral or not harmful and/or they do not interact with an AED or other modern epilepsy treatments. *Second*, their effect is harmful or detrimental to the patient because of primary/secondary effects or undesired interactions. *Third*, they are not effective as an AED, but they do promote general health. *Fourth*, their effect is unknown, and, therefore, most likely risky. *Fifth*, they are effective as an AED.

CONCLUSION

Because of the wide range of CAM effects, patients and medical providers need to discuss openly the use of CAMs in the acute and chronic treatment of epilepsy. Widespread non-adherence to evidence-based epilepsy treatments can be attributed to inadequate education, AED unavailability, insufficient resources, cultural beliefs, and wide use of CAMs.

A comprehensive epilepsy education program, along with improved access to evidence-based AEDs, appears to be the initial step to change non-adherent behaviors and to close the epilepsy treatment gap of non-adherence to prescribed evidence-based anti-convulsant medications and other therapies [Meinardi et al, 2001].

At the same time, clinical translational research needs to be promoted to determine newer specific and alternative therapies for epilepsy, some of which may prove to be CAMs currently in use at the present time.

REFERENCES

AAN. Report of the Quality Standards Subcommittee and Therapeutics and Technology Assessment Subcommittee of the American Academy of Neurology and American Epilepsy Society (2009) Practice Parameter update: Management issues for women with epilepsy—focus on pregnancy (an evidence-based review): Vitamin K, folic acid, blood levels, and breastfeeding. *Epilepsia*. 50(5):1247-55.

Ahola-Erkkilä S, Carroll C, Peltola-Mjösund K, Tulkki V, Mattila I, Seppänen-Laakso T, et al.(2010) Ketogenic diet slows down mitochondrial myopathy progression in mice. *Human Mol. Genet.* Feb. 17, (e-pub ahead of print).

de Almeida ER, Rafael KR, Couto GB, Ishigami AB.(2009) Anxiolytic and anticonvulsant effects on mice of flavonoids, linalool, and alpha-tocopherol presents in the extract of leaves of Cissus sicyoides L.(Vitaceae). *J. Biomed .Biotechnol*;274740.

Awad R, Ahmed F, Bourbonnais-Spear N, Mullally M, Ta CA, Tang A, et al. (2009) Ethnopharmacology of Q'eqchi' Maya antiepileptic and anxiolytic plants: effects on the GABAergic system. *J. Ethnopharmacol*, 125(2):257-64.

Barnes PM, Powell-Griner E, JcFann K, Nahin RL.(2004) *Complementary and alternative medicine use among adults*: United States. Adv. Data;343:1-19.

Bergen DC (1998) Preventable neurological diseases worldwide. *Neuroepidemiolog*, 17(2):67-73.

Bum EN, Taiwe GS, Nkainsa LA, Moto FC, Seke Etet PF, Hiana IR, et al (2009) Validation of anticonvulsant and sedative activity of six medicinal plants. *Epilepsy Behav*, 14(3):454-8.

Cheuk DKL,Wong V. Acupuncture for epilepsy. *Cochrane Database of Systematic Reviews* 2008, Issue 4. Art. No.: CD005062. DOI: 10.1002/14651858.CD005062.pub3.

Collings JA (1994) International differences in psychosocial well-being: a comparative study of adults with epilepsy in three countries. *Seizure*, 3:183-190.

Devinsky O, Cramer JA (1993) Introduction: Quality of Life in Epilepsy *Epilepsia*, 34(suppl 4):1-3.

Dodrill CB (1993) *Historical perspectives and future directions.* In: The treatment of epilepsy: principles and practices. Edited by Elaine Wyllie. Philadelphia, Lea and Febiger, 1129-1132.

Durón R, Medina MT, Boyd D, Stansbury J.(2001) *Antropología de las epilepsias.* In: Medina, Chávez, Chinchilla and Gracia Eds. Las Epilepsias en Centroamérica. Scancolor: Tegucigalpa, 229-235.

Durón R, Medina MT, Holden K, Ramírez F, et al. (2001) Estudio sobre el cumplimiento del tratamiento por los pacientes epilépticos del Hospital Escuela. *Rev. Med. Hond.* 69(4).

Durón RM, Medina MT, Nicolás O, Varela FE, Ramírez F, Battle SJ, Thompson A, Rodríguez LC, Oseguera C, Aguilar-Estrada RL, Pietsch-Escueta S, Collins JS, Holden

KR (2009) Adherence and complementary and alternative medicine use among Honduran people with epilepsy. *Epilepsy Behav*, 14(4):645-50.

Elferink JG (1999) *Epilepsy in the ancient cultures of America* (I). International Epilepsy News. Netherlands: International Bureau for Epilepsy, 137:5-8.

Freeman JM, Vining EP, Kossoff EH, Pyzik PL, Ye X, Goodman SN (2009) A blinded, crossover study of the efficacy of the ketogenic diet. *Epilepsia*, 50(2):322-5.

Grundmann O, Wang J, McGregor GP, Butterweck V (2008) Anxiolytic activity of a phytochemically characterized Passiflora incarnate extract is mediated via the GABAergic system. *Planta Med*, 74(15):1769-73.

Heidari MR, Dadollahi Z, Mehrabani M, Mehrabi H, Pourzadeh-Hosseini M, Behravan E, et al(2009) Study of antiseizure effects of Matricaria recutita extract in mice. *Ann. N. Y. Acad. Sci*,1171:300-4.

Jilek-Aall L, Jilek M, Kaaya J, Mkombachepa L, Hillary K(1997) Psychosocial study of epilepsy in Africa. *Soc. Sci. Med*, 45(5):783-95.

Jindal V, Ge A, Mansky PJ (2008) Safety and efficacy of acupuncture in children: a review of the evidence. *J. Pediatr Hematol. Oncol*, 30(6):431–42.

Kaiboriboon K, Guevara M, Alldredge BK (2009) Understanding herb and dietary supplement use in patients with epilepsy. *Epilepsia*, 50:1927-32.

Kossoff EH, Dorward JL, Molinero MR, Holden KR (2008) The modified Atkins diet: A potential treatment for developing countries. *Epilepsia*, 49:1646-47.

Lai CW, YH Lai (1991) History of epilepsy in chinese traditional medicine. *Epilepsia*, 32(3):299-302.

Li Q, Chen X, He L, Zhou D. Traditional Chinese medicine for epilepsy. Cochrane Database of Systematic Reviews 2009, Issue 3. Art. No.: CD006454. DOI: 10.1002/14651858. CD006454.pub2.

Lundgren T, Dahl J, Yardi N, Melin L (2008) Acceptance and commitment therapy and yoga for drug-refractory epilepsy: a randomized controlled trial. *Epilepsy and Behavior*, 13:102–8.

Medina MT, Durón RM, Martínez L, Osorio JR, Estrada AL, Zúniga C, Cartagena D, Collins JS, Holden KR (2005) Prevalence, incidence, and etiology of epilepsies in rural Honduras: the Salamá study. *Epilepsia* 46:124-131.

Meinardi H, Scott RA, Reiss, JWAS Sander (2001) ILAE Commission report. The treatment gap in epilepsy: the current situation and ways forward. *Epilepsia*, 42(1):136-149.

Neto AC, Netto JC, Pereira PS, Pereira AM, Taleb-Contini SH, França SC, et al (2009) The role of polar phytocomplexes on anticonvulsant effects of leaf extracts of Lippia alba (Mill.) N.E. Brown chemotypes. *J. Pharm. Pharmacol*, 61(7):933-9.

National Library of Medicine (NLM). MedlinePlus. Drugs and supplements. All drugs and supplements.Accessed   03/10/2010a.   Available   from: http://www.nlm.nih.gov/ medlineplus/druginfo/herb

National Library of Medicine (NLM). Dietary Supplements Labels Database. Accessed 03/10/2010b. Available from: http://dietarysupplements.nlm.nih.gov/dietary/herbIngred. jsp.

Osuntokun B (1977) *Epilepsy in the African Continent*. In: Penry JK Ed. Epilepsy, The Eighth International Symposium, New York: Raven Press;:365-378.

Pal SK, Sharma K, Prabhakar S, Pathak A.(2008) Psychosocial, demographic, and treatment-seeking strategic behavior, including faith healing practices, among patients with epilepsy in northwest India. *Epilepsy Behav*, 13(2):323-32.

Ramaratnam S, Baker GA, Goldstein LH. *Psychological treatments for epilepsy*. Cochrane Database Syst. Rev. 2001;4:CD002029.

Samuels N, Finkelstein Y, Singer SR, Oberbaum M.(2008) Herbal medicine and epilepsy: proconvulsive effects and interactions with antiepileptic drugs. *Epilepsia*, 49(3):373-80.

Singh D, Goel RK(2009) Anticonvulsant effect of Ficus religiosa: role of serotonergic pathways. *J. Ethnopharmacol*, 123(2):330-4.

Tyagi A, Delanty N (2003) Herbal remedies, dietary supplements, and seizures. *Epilepsia* 44(2):228-35.

Varela F, Nicolás O, Durón R, Medina MT (2002) Aspectos antropológicos y culturales que inciden en la determinación de la prevalencia de las epilepsias en la etnia miskita de Honduras. *Rev. Med. Hond*, 70:9-14.

Vining EP(2008) Long-term health consequences of epilepsy diet treatments. *Epilepsia* 49(Suppl 8):27-9.

Wong M (2010) Herbs and spices: Unexpected sources of antiepileptogenic drug treatments? *Epilepsy Currents*, 10:21-23.Wu Z, Xu Q, Zhang L, Kong D, Ma R, Wang L (2009) Protective effect of resveratrol against kainate-induced temporal lobe epilepsy in rats. *Neurochem. Res*,34 (8):1393-400.

Yardi N (2001) Yoga for control of epilepsy. *Seizure*,10: 7–12.

INDEX

J

K

L

M

T